SECURING HEALTH IN SOUTHEAST ASIA

FEBRUARY 2025

ASIAN DEVELOPMENT BANK

ADB

6 ADB Avenue, Mandaluyong City, 1550 Metro Manila, Philippines
Tel +63 2 8632 4444; Fax +63 2 8636 2444
www.adb.org

ISBN 978-92-9277-208-6 (print); 978-92-9277-209-3 (PDF); 978-92-9277-210-9 (ebook)
Publication Stock No. TCS250070
DOI: http://dx.doi.org/10.22617/TCS250070

Notes:
In this publication, "$" refers to United States dollars.
ADB recognizes "China" as the People's Republic of China and "Laos" as the Lao People's Democratic Republic.

Cover design by Mike Cortes.

CONTENTS

Appendixes

TABLES AND FIGURE

Tables

Figure

FOREWORD

During the coronavirus disease (COVID-19) pandemic, the Asian Development Bank (ADB) was placed in the unique position of working closely with national and local governments, private sector entities, academic and medical communities, and other groups and institutions in Southeast Asia as they responded to an unprecedented public health crisis.

Within weeks of the announcement of a global pandemic, ADB had put together a fund of $20 billion to support programs across its developing member countries (DMCs), particularly in the form of health sector emergency assistance grants and loans and contingent disaster financing. It also supported private sector responses through direct financing, working capital support, and trade and supply chain finance. ADB also approved the $9 billion Asia Pacific Vaccine Access Facility in December 2020 to support DMCs in providing safe, equitable, and effective COVID-19 vaccines.

DMCs in Southeast Asia were among the Asia Pacific Vaccine Access Facility beneficiaries, beginning with the Philippines and Indonesia in March 2021. However, despite the countries' efforts, vaccination rollout in the region was faced with delays and numerous challenges, many relating to inequity and hesitancy. In the hope of supporting vaccination programs, a technical assistance (TA) facility was established to cover seven DMCs: Cambodia, Indonesia, the Lao People's Democratic Republic, the Philippines, Thailand, Timor-Leste, and Viet Nam. Entitled "Supporting Enhanced COVID-19 Vaccination and Post-COVID-19 Health Security Response in Southeast Asia" (TA 6767), this facility aimed to support various aspects of vaccination and other COVID-related programs including logistics, regulation, contingency planning, information systems, regional health security, and the sharing of best practices.

This publication compiles some of the lessons learned from our partners in the region during this year-long engagement and offers insights into the process of trying to accomplish all the stated goals of the TA. Assembled and drafted by national and regional experts, the book's chapters zoom into different aspects of vaccination, from public–private partnerships and communication to pharmacovigilance and digitization, that have proven to be decisive in shaping the successes met and challenges faced by the DMCs. While by no means comprehensive in scope or timeframe, these chapters nonetheless provide contemporary, grounded accounts of public health in practice. As such, they can be in conversation with other such efforts in the region, as well as scholarly analyses of the same topics around the world.

As this book was being prepared, 3 years after COVID-19 shut down much of Southeast Asia, the pandemic is receding from view, and governments have lifted exceptional measures that consider the viral outbreak a public health emergency. Nonetheless, COVID-19 continues to affect people around the world, and the issues identified in this book remain salient for health programs in general, from countering vaccine hesitancy to digitizing health information systems.

We hope the chapters of this book will serve as reminders of the complex challenges governments and societies faced with COVID-19 and as a reference for how to prepare for future pandemics and work toward more resilient and responsive health systems in the region.

Eduardo Banzon
Director
Human and Social Development Sector Office
Sectors Group

ACKNOWLEDGMENTS

This publication is a collaboration among public health advocates across Southeast Asia.

Eduardo Banzon, director, Human and Social Development Sector Office, ADB, spearheaded its creation as project team leader.

This publication is made possible with the support of Ramesh Subramaniam, director general and Group Chief, Sectors Group, ADB (SG-ADB); Sungsup Ra, former deputy director general and deputy group chief, SG-ADB; Ayako Inagaki, senior director, Human and Social Development Sector Office, ADB; and Karin Schelzig, director, Human and Social Development Sector Office, ADB.

Alexo Esperato and Shekinah Wenceslao contributed greatly in streamlining the logistical and organizational aspects of the project. Randy Dacanay, Liza Tabora, and Sarah Cueno provided methodical oversight as the project's coordinating team.

Gideon Lasco and Vincen Gregory Yu served as editors and supplementary writers of the publication. Editorial support was also provided by Shekinah Wenceslao, Marc Miranda, Randy Dacanay, and Liza Tabora.

Chapter 1 was built on existing and previous work by Sam Sternin (Cambodia), Bouathep Phoumindr (Lao People's Democratic Republic [Lao PDR]), Manivone Thikeo (Lao PDR), Khanchit Limpakarnjanarat (Thailand), Nguyen Thi Hong Tu (Viet Nam), Jeremy Gorospe (Philippines), and Rabiah al Adawiyah (Indonesia). Likewise, Chapter 2 made use of existing work by Abigail Generalia, Duong Minh Duoc (Viet Nam), Cecil Behino (Philippines), Rahmat Hidayat Efendi (Indonesia), and Worapon Rattanawarawong (Thailand). Chapter 3 was written by Raymond Sarmiento, Chapter 4 by Kyi Thar, and Chapter 5 by Swee Kheng Khor.

Finally, Ly Sovann (Ministry of Health, Cambodia); Bounserth Keoprasith (Ministry of Health, Lao PDR), Rattanaxay Phetsouvanh (Ministry of Health, Lao PDR), Vichan Pawun (Ministry of Public Health, Thailand), Chaninan Sonthichai (Ministry of Public Health, Thailand), and Beverly Ho (Philippines) each lent their valuable insights, expertise, and time to the interviews that appear in the final sections of this publication.

ABBREVIATIONS

ADB	Asian Development Bank
ADR	adverse drug reaction
AEFI	adverse events following immunization
ASEAN	Association of Southeast Asian Nations
DAV	Drug Administration Viet Nam
DDF	Department of Drugs and Food, Cambodia
DMC	developing member country
DOH	Department of Health
eHAC	Electronic Health Alert Card
FDA	Food and Drug Administration
FDD	Food and Drug Department, Lao People's Democratic Republic
GBT	Global Benchmarking Tool
GMP	Good Manufacturing Practices
HNAP	Health National Adaptation Plan of the Lao People's Democratic Republic
HSI	health security intervention
IPC	Institut Pasteur Cambodia
LGU	local government unit in the Philippines
MOH	Ministry of Health
MRA-GMP	mutual recognition arrangement on good manufacturing practice inspection
NADFC	National Agency of Drug and Food Control
NHSO	National Health Security Office, Thailand
NIIS	National Immunization Information System of Viet Nam
NRA	national regulatory authority
POM	provincial health departments in Indonesia
PPP	public–private partnership
SAGE	WHO Strategic Advisory Group of Experts
SARS	Severe Acute Respiratory Syndrome
SDG	Sustainable Development Goal
SMILE	Sistem Monitoring Imunisasi dan Logistik Secara Elektronik
T3	Test, Trace, Treat
TA	technical assistance
UNDP	United Nations Development Programme
UNICEF	United Nations Children's Fund
VIMS	Vaccine Information Management System of the Philippines
VIS	vaccine information system

EXECUTIVE SUMMARY

This publication is a product of the Supporting Enhanced COVID-19 Vaccination and Post-COVID-19 Health Security Response in Southeast Asia (SECURE) technical facility of the Asia Development Bank (Technical Assistance [TA] 6767), which was established to support various aspects of vaccination and other coronavirus disease (COVID-19) programs, including logistics, regulation, contingency planning, information systems, and regional health security. In the course of SECURE's collaboration throughout the pandemic with seven developing member countries (DMCs)—Cambodia, Indonesia, the Lao People's Democratic Republic (Lao PDR), the Philippines, Thailand, Timor-Leste, and Viet Nam—the need to learn and document lessons from this unique moment in public health was recognized and found shape and form in this publication with the help of experts and partners from all the seven countries. The publication is not meant to offer an exhaustive discussion of the topics raised or to analyze each country according to each of those topics. However, its five chapters shed light on some aspects of vaccination programs that were crucial in shaping the outcomes of some of the DMCs' pandemic response, thereby contributing to the broader literature.

The first chapter, Implementing COVID-19 Vaccination Programs, provides a brief overview of the vaccination programs in Cambodia, Indonesia, the Lao PDR, the Philippines, Thailand, and Viet Nam, as recounted by people intimately involved in their implementation. The chapter highlights the strengths and best practices of each country and points out the challenges and opportunities for further improvement of these programs. Aside from affirming the need to prioritize the topics addressed in the succeeding chapters, it recommends sustained investments in health and a targeted approach that accounts for the geographic, demographic, socioeconomic, and cultural diversity within DMCs.

The second chapter, Communicating Vaccines and Countering Hesitancy, focuses on the much-discussed but poorly understood phenomenon of vaccine hesitancy. It discusses its consequences in the region and offers recommendations, from identifying and mapping stakeholders to communicating more effectively with target audiences. At the heart of this chapter is the recognition and call to action that, beyond the labor of developing, procuring, and distributing vaccines, public health institutions should strive to foster an enabling environment for people to accept those vaccines. This includes addressing their context-specific concerns, mapping and forging strong partnerships with stakeholders, and making vaccination more convenient.

The third chapter, Digitizing Vaccine Information Systems, discusses how governments might integrate technologies into various pandemic-related processes, including surveillance, testing, contact tracing, and quarantine. Recognized as one of the building blocks of health systems, health information systems have always been a project for governments, but the pandemic has heightened the need for their implementation while also ushering in the adoption of various digital technologies such as QR codes and digital prescriptions. This chapter highlights the ways in which digital technologies were adopted as part of health systems and how they might be further adopted as part of recovery from the pandemic. It concludes by calling for robust investment in widely accessible, user-friendly, interoperable, and secure digital infrastructure, as well as regional standardization.

The fourth chapter, Improving Pharmacovigilance, zeroes in on regulatory systems. Given the scale of the pandemic and the record-breaking speed of vaccine development, regulatory systems around the world struggled to streamline or expedite regulatory processes without compromising standards for safety and efficacy. This chapter discusses how Cambodia, Indonesia, the Lao PDR, the Philippines, Thailand, Timor-Leste, and Viet Nam improved and promoted their pharmacovigilance (PV) systems during the pandemic and cites some recommendations for how to improve existing systems from transparent, responsive feedback mechanisms to harmonizing PV systems at the regional level.

Finally, the fifth chapter, Mobilizing Public–Private Partnerships, highlights the role of the private sector, as well as the opportunities and challenges of entering public–private partnerships (PPPs), not just in vaccination programs but in health systems more broadly. Over the past decade, governments in the region have looked at PPPs as drivers of economic stimulus and recovery, but the glaring inequities between public and private health care in many DMCs have translated to public sector concerns over the fairness of such arrangements. With profound impacts on both public and private sectors–from supply chains to human resources–the pandemic has tested some of the assumptions about PPPs, even as it reanimated the need to consider alternative strategies to finance health care infrastructure and services, including private sector involvement. This chapter begins with single-country analyses of six DMCs in the region, identifying particular challenges and common patterns, and concludes by integrating recommendations for how fairer, more effective PPPs can be realized, including the establishment of clear policy frameworks and the need for the private sector to recognize inclusive development as a guiding principle in its engagements in public health.

CHAPTER 1

Implementing COVID-19 Vaccination Programs

KEY POINTS

- Despite financial and structural constraints, Cambodia, Indonesia, the Lao People's Democratic Republic, the Philippines, Thailand, and Viet Nam achieved remarkable successes in some aspects of their pandemic response, setting examples for the rest of the world.
- On the vaccine supply side, best practices included vaccine diplomacy involving proactive procurement strategy, bilateral relationships, diversified vaccine portfolios, and strengthened research and development for manufacturing vaccines.
- As for vaccine distribution and demand, these practices included comprehensive planning, feedback mechanisms, digital technologies, addressing and collaborations. with the private sector.

This chapter looks into the implementation of coronavirus disease (COVID-19) vaccination programs in six Asian Development Bank (ADB) developing member countries (DMCs), —Cambodia, Indonesia, the Lao People's Democratic Republic (Lao PDR), the Philippines, Thailand, and Viet Nam. Most, if not all, of these countries faced profound challenges in securing vaccine supplies on top of structural health issues. For example, especially in its rural parts, Cambodia had a health workforce density that was well below the average for low- and middle-income countries (only 0.2 doctors and 0.7 nurses per 1,000 people, compared to the recommended average of 0.6 doctors and 1.3 nurses per 1,000 people).[1] On the other hand, the Philippines had long struggled with widespread inadequacies in its public health system, even with the upcoming implementation of a universal health care law.

These constraints notwithstanding, the six DMCs made significant strides in vaccinating their respective populations against COVID-19 (with some countries admittedly faring better than others). By April 2021, for instance, only around 4 months since vaccinations started around the world, Indonesia had already administered some 18.5 million doses to its population, reportedly making it the 12th largest implementation program worldwide—an all

[1] Organisation for Economic Co-operation and Development (OECD) and World Health Organization (WHO). 2020. *Health at a Glance: Asia/Pacific 2020: Measuring Progress towards Universal Health Coverage.* https://doi.org/10.1787/26b007cd-en.

the more remarkable achievement when one considers the country's archipelagic geography.[2] Cambodia has managed to avoid terrible outcomes during the pandemic: the country has credited its vaccination program as part of its "success" in minimizing its death toll (over 3,000 deaths as of June 2023).[3]

So, how exactly did these DMCs fare in terms of their respective vaccination programs, and what lessons can be gleaned from their experiences? This chapter outlines the collective best practices of those vaccination programs, examining how governments procured and rolled out the vaccines, fostered international and national partnerships to increase supply and hasten uptake, and tackled obstacles to vaccine acceptance from the lack of relevant technologies to the spread of misinformation. In embarking on this analysis, this chapter thus allows for an identification of points of improvement with regard to vaccination programs and vaccine-related policies not only in these DMCs but also in countries that have endured similar circumstances throughout the pandemic (Table 1).

Table 1: Summary of Vaccination Programs

Country	Vaccine Supply	Vaccine Distribution and Demand
Cambodia	**Bilateral negotiations** with manufacturers to supply vaccines in advance of WHO and stringent regulatory authority approvals	**Campaign delivery** with rapid feedback and adjustment to maximize vaccine coverage **Large workforce to administer vaccines** **Multilingual risk communications**, including minority languages
Indonesia	**Diversified portfolio of eligible vaccines**—regulatory approval for 10 different vaccines	**Comprehensive planning**, including funding programs by the government and private sector, early identification of priority populations for vaccination, waste management **Accessible and convenient vaccination points** **Digital health innovations** to monitor vaccine stocks
Lao People's Democratic Republic	**Bilateral relations** with major vaccine-manufacturing countries	**Bilateral relations** with suppliers of cold chain and logistical equipment **Campaign style** with extensive use of multimedia
Philippines	**Tripartite agreements** between governments, private companies, and manufacturers	**Private sector involvement** in rollout and communications efforts
Thailand	**Strengthening R&D for manufacturing vaccines**	**Compensating adverse events** to bolster people's trust
Viet Nam	**Strengthening R&D for manufacturing vaccines**	**Large workforce to administer vaccines** **Epidemiological assessments** to identify under-vaccinated groups and geographies

R&D = research and development; WHO = World Health Organization.

[2] B. Arifin and T. Anas. 2021. Lessons Learned from COVID-19 Vaccination in Indonesia: Experiences, Challenges, and Opportunities. *Human Vaccines & Immunotherapeutics*. 17 (11). pp. 2898–2906. https://doi.org/10.1080/21645515.2021.1975450.

[3] Our World in Data. *Coronavirus (COVID-19) Deaths*. https://ourworldindata.org/covid-deaths.

Vaccine Diplomacy and Proactive Procurement Strategies

The first best practice is vaccine diplomacy, which involves a proactive procurement strategy. This was most crucial during the first 2 years of the pandemic, when, as with many developing countries, none of the five DMCs had mechanisms to manufacture the vaccines locally and were therefore dependent on international sources, including the World Health Organization (WHO) COVAX Facility.

In the case of Cambodia, for instance, rather than wait for donations with unclear delivery timelines, the government negotiated directly with vaccine manufacturers and paid competitive prices to ensure rapid delivery. Reaching out to manufacturers in the People's Republic of China (PRC) Sinovac and Sinopharm long before their vaccines received regulatory approval from WHO, the country was able to source a sufficient number of doses, while many countries continued waiting for delayed deliveries under bilateral or multilateral agreements. This proved prudent for the country, which started its COVID-19 vaccination campaign as early as February 2021, just as it was experiencing its first major domestic outbreaks. This swiftness of governmental action could also be credited for how the country not only emerged as one of the countries with the highest levels of coverage for first and second doses by mid-2021 but also one of the first countries to introduce a third booster dose in the fall of 2021.

Diplomatic ties were also crucial to the vaccination experience of the Lao PDR. In mid-2021, as the Delta variant swept across the country while its vaccine supply remained inadequate,[4] the Government of the Lao PDR was able to rely on the neighboring PRC for swift supplies of Sinopharm vaccines, over four million doses of which were delivered to the country in 6 months.[5] These vaccine deliveries could be credited for mitigating the potential impact of the deadly variant during this particular surge in the country. Additionally, the Lao PDR's ties with Japan also resulted in the latter providing the former with refrigerated vaccine transport vehicles, which were necessary to improve vaccine access to the country's many remote, mountainous, and highly inaccessible communities.[6]

Indonesia also had the benefit of proactive leadership and flexible policies involving vaccinations during these crucial first 2 years. As early as the end of 2020, as the first vaccinations were rolled out in the United States (US) and the United Kingdom, the Government of Indonesia had already secured procurement agreements with many international manufacturers. Pivotal to the country's whole-of-government approach was the implementation of the Vaccination Allocation Plan (VAP) decreed by Presidential Regulation No. 99/2020, as amended by Presidential Regulation No. 14/2021, which provided specific plans on the whole vaccination strategy, from prioritization and procurement to waste

---

4 S. Strangio. 2021. Laos Tightens COVID-19 Restrictions as Infections Reach New Peak. *The Diplomat.* 22 September. https://thediplomat.com/2021/09/laos-tightens-covid-19-restrictions-as-infections-reach-new-peak/.

5 L. Phonevilay. 2021. China Donates Another Million Doses of Covid-19 Vaccines to Laos. *The Laotian Times,* 13 October. https://laotiantimes.com/2021/10/13/china-donates-another-million-doses-of-covid-19-vaccine-to-laos/.

6 UNICEF Lao PDR. 2023. *Lao PDR to Use Refrigerated Vaccine Transport Vehicles to Expand Immunization Coverage in Rural Areas.* 9 January. https://www.unicef.org/laos/press-releases/lao-pdr-use-refrigerated-vaccine-transport-vehicles-expand-immunization-coverage?gad=1&gclid=Cj0KCQjw7uSkBhDGARIsAMCZNJv6_hRk1KvlnheLlZCwLjeF2m7yv42giE_t2v6j6knsBxEcFIklpPwaAiXWEALw_wcB.

management. The VAP consisted of government- and employer-funded programs. The government-funded program sought to vaccinate 181.5 million Indonesians free of charge, while the employer-funded program accelerated vaccination coverage by allowing business entities to purchase vaccines from Bio Farma or other organizations authorized by the Minister of Health, to vaccinate employees and their families free of charge.[7]

This multipronged strategy thus enabled Indonesia to vaccinate over 1.1 million people with two doses at the end of the first quarter of 2021.[8] By the end of that year, the country had received more than 470 million doses of the COVID-19 vaccines and permitted the use of 10 brands, including those of Sinovac, AstraZeneca, Sinopharm, Moderna, Pfizer, Novavax, Sputnik V, Janssen, Convidencia, and Zifivax.[9]

Aggressive, Multisectoral Vaccine Rollout

A proactive procurement strategy had to be accompanied by an aggressive rollout system. This is the second-best practice—countries enjoining all sectors and deploying all available resources to implement the vaccination programs as quickly and widely as possible.

Cambodia demonstrated the virtues of a campaign-style implementation system, which targeted both priority populations (older people and frontline workers) as well as priority geographies (COVID-19 hotspots) to ensure that vaccines were easily accessible to those at greatest risk. This vaccine delivery strategy was then regularly updated based on the experience gained on the ground, for example, by adding additional vaccine delivery points and adopting more mobile delivery mechanisms for hard-to-reach populations. Indonesia also realized the value of a more accessible and flexible delivery system. The acceleration of its vaccination implementation strategy was in part made possible by using strategic public places (with drive-through and walk-in options), public and private offices, and engaging private sectors to implement the vaccination.[10] Meanwhile, the Lao PDR's campaign-style implementation and promotion, developed in partnership with the United Nations Children's Fund (UNICEF), involved utilizing all forms of media to raise awareness, including posters and banners, radio spots, social media content, and even music videos.[11]

Cambodia and Viet Nam both demonstrated that effective rollouts involve mobilizing large numbers of implementors, from health workers and community volunteers to even the armed forces—a method similarly adopted by Indonesia, where the TNI/POLRI (Indonesian National Armed Forces) played a supporting role to health workers in implementing

---

7 This figure was determined by taking the total population aged over 18 (188.7 million) and excluding 7.2 million people for whom vaccines were yet to be proven safe and efficacious, such as pregnant women.

8 Government of Indonesia, Office of Assistant to Deputy Cabinet Secretary for State Documents & Translation. 2021. *COVID-19 Task Force: Continue to Build Cooperation in Reducing COVID-19 Cases.* 24 May. https://setkab.go.id/en/covid-19-task-force-continue-to-build-cooperation-in-reducing-covid-19-cases/.

9 United Nations Office for the Coordination of Humanitarian Affairs (OCHA). 2022. *Situation Update: Response to COVID-19 in Indonesia.* 5 January. https://reliefweb.int/report/indonesia/situation-update-response-covid-19-indonesia-5-january-2022.

10 Y. Mahendradhata et al. 2021. The Capacity of the Indonesian Healthcare system to Respond to COVID-19. *Frontiers in Public Health* 9. 649819. https://www.frontiersin.org/articles/10.3389/fpubh.2021.649819/full.

11 UNICEF. 2021. *UNICEF Lao People's Democratic Republic Country Office Annual Report 2021.* https://www.unicef.org/reports/country-regional-divisional-annual-reports-2021/Lao-Peoples-Democratic-Republic.

vaccinations, especially workers in remote parts of the country.[12] Additionally, the value of evolving feedback was also recognized by these countries. In Cambodia, for example, regular analysis of vaccination data by the Ministry of Health enabled the identification of pockets of low coverage, which could then be prioritized for follow-up. Viet Nam, meanwhile, also constantly adjusted its strategy based on epidemiological developments to focus on evolving notions of "high-risk" populations and areas.

Digitalization of Vaccination Campaigns

The third best practice (discussed further in Chapter 3) involves embracing technology: digitizing the processes related to the vaccination campaign. Indonesia's high coverage rate could be attributed to the concerted efforts of multiple major institutions in working toward a transformative digitalization process spearheaded by the Ministry of Health. Two important results of these efforts were the One Data health information system and PeduliLindungi application, real-time digital systems to monitor vaccine stocks and distribution, and the PCare application that enabled frontline health workers to submit vaccination data more efficiently into One Data.

It is important to note that in Indonesia, integrating health data and information systems has always been a challenge, with nearly 270 million people spread across 34 provinces and 541 districts. This geographical situation is further compounded by the limited integration between various levels of public and private information systems, making work more difficult for health workers tasked to manage similar data across multiple applications on a daily basis, sometimes by relying on manual systems in the face of failing digital ones.[13]

Initiated in 2014 but fully realized only during the pandemic, One Data (or Satu Data Indonesia) was Indonesia's solution to a robust process of data collection, processing, analysis, and dissemination necessary to produce measurable information for a responsive and successful COVID-19 surveillance system—a one-stop shop of sorts for synthesizing COVID-19-related data in the country (footnote 13). PeduliLindungi is another mobile app developed by the Ministry of Telecommunication and Informatics, providing information to relevant government agencies carrying out contact tracing, akin to the United Kingdom's Bluetooth-enabled "track and trace" application. Quite distinctly, PeduliLindungi relied on community participation to share and register location data while also providing users with information if they were in red zones (i.e., areas with high cases of COVID-19). The information in this app was then linked to a central information system that also connected to One Data.[14]

---

12 D. Rochmyaningsih. 2022. How Indonesia Got Vaccinated. *GAVI*. 2 June. https://www.gavi.org/vaccineswork/how-indonesia-got-vaccinated.

13 Partnership for Australia-Indonesia Centre. 2021. One Data: COVID-19, Health Data Connectivity and Integration in Indonesia–A Case Study of Yogyakarta. *The Australia-Indonesia Centre*. 4 August. https://pair.australiaindonesiacentre.org/featured/one-data-covid-19-health-data-connectivity-and-integration-in-indonesia-a-case-study-of-yogyakarta/.

14 D. N. Aisyah et al. 2022. Building on Health Security Capacities in Indonesia: Lessons Learned from the COVID-19 Pandemic Responses and Challenges. *Zoonoses and Public Health*. 69 (6). pp. 757–767. https://onlinelibrary.wiley.com/doi/epdf/10.1111/zph.12976.

Most significant to the vaccination program of the country, however, was SMILE (System Information for Immunisation Logistic, or, in Bahasa, Sistem Monitoring Imunisasi dan Logistik Secara Elektronik). This app was developed to enable real-time visibility of vaccine cold chain logistics and digitize stock supplies and storage temperature across vaccine cold chain points. By the end of 2021, SMILE was already effectively in use in 18 provinces.

SMILE was first implemented in 2018, but it was only scaled up during the pandemic, where a target of 10,000 facilities in 5 years was set. SMILE itself consists of a mobile app for cold chain handlers, a web interface for data storage, and a digital temperature logger that automatically monitors the storage temperature of vaccines to ensure the quality of vaccines that are delivered. With the analytics system on the SMILE web interface, health workers can check whether vaccines are overstocked, falling short of the prescribed levels, or completely stocked out, allowing data to be available even from the most remote locations. Suffice it to say, the implementation of SMILE contributed to the operational efficiencies and addressed inequities in vaccine coverage across the country. The application combined technology, systematic record-keeping practices, and a network of trained personnel to support health workers in addressing huge inequities in vaccine coverage that contribute to overstocking and stock-outs of vaccines in storage centers.

Private Sector Partnerships

A fourth best practice is partnering with the private sector (Chapter 5 has a more extended discussion). This was most evident in the Philippines, where public health facilities and resources had long been ill-equipped to handle even the pre-pandemic health situation in the country. While the Government of the Philippines had been implementing national vaccination for many years, it never did so at anywhere near the scale that COVID-19 demanded nor at the speed required to achieve population protection. It could not accommodate the sophisticated logistic requirements of storing and transporting eight vaccine platforms with different temperature requirements. It also could not reprogram the national budget quickly enough to accommodate those requirements.

Recognizing its sheer inability to cope with the extraordinary strains of the pandemic on the Philippines' health system, the government thus sought out the help of the country's private sector (e.g., private companies and corporations), which had the scale of human resources and the reach across the country to quickly implement mass vaccinations. Unlike the national government, the private sector could easily reprogram its budget and make business decisions to invest in technologies and equipment, had a more diverse pool of expertise that could be easily tapped based on the need at the time, and had contributors that already mostly provided their knowledge and expertise to the state pro bono.

Thus, the Task Force Test, Trace, Treat (T3) private sector consortium was created from this partnership; a response initially channeled through conglomerates in the Philippines to augment the government's response to COVID-19. As demand for the COVID-19 response broadened, more companies joined Task Force T3 and offered what they could to help the country. Rival companies started working together, competitors brainstormed to provide great ideas, and people from different sides and different fields of expertise sat together and listened to each other.

For example, the Chief Sustainability Officer from the fast-food chain Jollibee Foods Corporation provided the strategy and roadmap on how to achieve the goal of having high vaccine coverage by Christmas of 2021, focusing the company's efforts in the National Capital Region and its adjacent provinces where people outside the country usually entered via international flights in Manila. A supply chain expert was brought in by ADB to help plan and monitor the logistics and trace the vaccines. Meanwhile, the managing director of McDonald's Philippines worked closely with the Health Promotions Bureau of the Department of Health (DOH) to provide strategic and tailored information about COVID-19 and vaccines, as well as to debunk fake news spreading across social media and to increase vaccine acceptance.

To date, Task Force T3 is the biggest public–private coalition the country has seen. It has mobilized the private sector resources, expertise, and network to help in the COVID-19 response. The initial assistance needed was to help increase the country's testing capacity from 4,500 tests per day. After its inception, Task Force T3 was able to increase the testing capacity to 34,000 tests per day in only a month and eventually up to 100,000 tests per day by building testing laboratories across the country and providing the necessary equipment.

Relevantly for this chapter, Task Force T3 managed to facilitate a one-of-a-kind tripartite agreement (i.e., between the government, private sector, and the manufacturer or supplier) for COVID-19 vaccines when vaccine manufacturers were allowed to sell only directly to governments. This enabled member conglomerates and companies of the task force to procure vaccines for their employees, their employees' dependents, and donate vaccines to the government. Their efforts did not stop there. The tripartite agreement allowed the country to substantially increase vaccine supply. However, the private sector did not stop at augmenting the vaccine supply. T3 extended its assistance throughout and across many dimensions of the vaccination rollout, from planning, logistics, distribution, communication, and actual inoculation. In all, this partnership provided the country a glimpse of what the most efficient public–private partnership (PPP) can achieve in advancing health outcomes at the most crucial moments.

Local Vaccine Research, Manufacturing, and Development

However, perhaps the very pinnacle of self-reliance in vaccinating an entire population can be seen in how some countries started developing their own COVID-19 vaccines rather than relying entirely on importations or donations from the COVAX facility. Although these efforts were ultimately unsuccessful in the timelines required, they nonetheless facilitated various elements—from research partnerships to manufacturing infrastructure—that have placed those countries in a better position to respond to future pandemics (even as the very availability of this option required pre-existing infrastructure).

Thailand provides an example of this best practice. In setting out to manufacture its local vaccines, the country gathered the academic sector, government research institutes, and private companies to embark on that goal based on the "Blueprint of Access to COVID Vaccine for Thailand" developed in 2021. In ensuring access to a vaccine for the entire population of Thailand, that blueprint not only considered advance market commitment, or purchasing vaccines from international manufacturers in advance and looking for opportunities for vaccine technology transfer, but also and more significantly, supporting domestic COVID-19 vaccine research and development.

This blueprint was successfully implemented, resulting in over 150 million doses of COVID-19 vaccine for Thai and non-Thai people who lived in the country by 2022. On the vaccine development front, two of the candidates (ChulaCov by Chulalongkorn University and NDP-HXP COVID-19 vaccine (HXP-GPOVac) by the Government Pharmaceutical Organization) made significant progress, culminating in the emergency use authorization for HXP-GPOVac in January 2024. Crucially, the National Vaccine Institute has continued supporting the establishment of vaccine infrastructure and encouraging sustainable research for future epidemic and vaccine security. The envisaged timeline to complete the necessary infrastructure for domestic COVID-19 vaccine production is 3 years.

Viet Nam, too, started developing its own vaccines. On 25 October 2022, Deputy Prime Minister Vu Duc Dam signed Decision 1286/QD-TTg to ensure vaccine supply for immunization until 2030. Setting out goals to master vaccine production technologies on a local scale, the program thus laid the groundwork for local COVID-19 vaccine manufacturing and trials. By the end of 2022, five vaccines were being researched and produced in Viet Nam, two of which were being researched and developed entirely by the country itself (Nano COVAX and Covivac), with two more using transferred technology from abroad (VBC-COV19-154 and Recombinant SARS-CoV-2 Spike Protein) and another one (Sputnik V) limited only to the processing and packaging as far as the country was concerned. To date, no locally manufactured vaccine is licensed for use by the Ministry of Health.

Combating Hesitancy and Misinformation

Finally, amid the implementation of their respective programs, the countries have also had to counter vaccine hesitancy and related misinformation online and offline. In this regard, some DMCs have been better than others at handling these hurdles through localized, culturally sensitive methods. Chapter 2 offers a more expansive discussion on this topic, offering principles on how to address vaccine hesitancy through communications and stakeholder engagement. Nonetheless, in line with the chapter's focus on providing an overview of program implementation, it is useful to briefly highlight examples of how the countries took toward combating vaccine-related hesitancy and misinformation.

In Cambodia, the Ministry of Health worked with UNICEF to prepare risk communications, including in minority languages, that were rolled out through community volunteers, mass media, and social media. Of note is that this proactive and nationally contextualized mechanism to combat misinformation involved monitoring social media to identify and address emerging narratives as deemed fit, thus resulting in extremely low levels of vaccine hesitancy in the country.

Indonesia, too, saw vaccine hesitancy as an obstacle to better vaccination coverage.[15] In a survey of 115,000 respondents in August 2020, 27% expressed hesitancy, citing concerns about vaccine safety, effectiveness, side effects, the country's health system preparedness,

[15] R. R. Nugraha et al. 2021. Accelerating Indonesian COVID-19 Vaccination Rollout: A Critical Task amid the Second Wave. *Tropical Medicine and Health*. 49. 76. https://tropmedhealth.biomedcentral.com/articles/10.1186/s41182-021-00367-3.

religious beliefs, and lack of education.[16] Subsequent surveys have yielded similar results.[17] A major issue involved the halal status of the vaccines, which was particularly relevant in light of the country's predominantly Muslim population. Thus, to address this concern around the time vaccinations were only starting, the Indonesian Ulama Council issued halal certifications for Sinovac and AstraZeneca vaccines, even as misinformation regarding the vaccine ingredients remained widespread online and off.

Meanwhile, one policy that may have helped Thailand allay people's fears about adverse effects, a major source of vaccine hesitancy, was its no-fault compensation scheme, in place even before the pandemic, that mirrored the approach implemented by over 20 other countries, including Viet Nam.[18] From the beginning of the vaccine rollout, the National Health Security Office (NHSO) made sure to inform people that they would be compensated if they experienced adverse effects from the vaccines by submitting claims for compensation at the hospitals where they got vaccinated or even in provincial health offices or NHSO regional offices.[19] While claims submissions still had to be scrutinized by a committee in each office, those claims that got approved entitled the recipient to a maximum of B400,000 for death or permanent disability, B240,000 for loss of an organ, and B100,000 for any injury or illness less severe than previously mentioned (footnote 19). From April 2021 to January 2022, the NHSO paid out around B1 billion in financial aid to over 9,000 approved claims.[20]

Of note were the four cases (one definite and three probable) of vaccine-induced immune thrombotic thrombocytonenia reported after the rollout of more than 35 million doses of ChAdOx1 nCoV-19 or Covishield in Thailand. Two of those cases resulted in death, which definitely contributed to hesitancy surrounding this brand of vaccines. This extremely rare adverse event was subsequently included in information presented to all potential recipients.[21]

Recommendations and Points for Improvement

Having identified best practices of the vaccination programs of the five DMCs have greatly advanced these programs and helped these countries to surmount the worst obstacles of the pandemic. However, there remains room for improvement, in handling the future evolution of COVID-19 with respect to vaccinations and in strengthening overall vaccination programs and vaccine-related policies.

---

16 Kementerian Kesehatan, ITAGI, UNICEF, and WHO, Survei Penerimaan Vaksin di Indonesia. Kemenkes RI, Jakarta, 2020.

17 A. Agustina et al. 2023. Overview of Knowledge and Acceptance of the DKI Jakarta Community on the Covid-19 Vaccination Program. *Journal of Medical and Health Studies*. 4 (2). pp. 53–58.

18 R. G. Mungwira et al. 2020. Global Landscape Analysis of No-Fault Compensation Programmes for Vaccine Injuries: A Review and Survey of Implementing Countries. *PLoS ONE* 15 (5). e0233334. https://doi.org/10.1371/journal.pone.0233334.

19 Government of Thailand, National Health Security Office. 2021. *A Guideline Issued for a COVID-19 Vaccine Side Effects Fund*. 20 May. https://eng.nhso.go.th/view/1/DescriptionNews/A-guideline-issued-for-a-COVID-19-vaccine-side-effects-fund/325/EN-US.

20 *Thai PBS World*. 2021. 927 Million Baht Paid to Over 8,000 People Suffering Side Effects from COVID Vaccinations. 27 December. https://eng.nhso.go.th/view/1/DescriptionNews/One-billion-baht-paid-to-COVID-19-vaccine-recipients-experiencing-side-effects-/409/EN-US.

21 S. A. Watcharananan et al. 2022. Rates, Types, and Associated Factors of Acute Adverse Effects After the First Dose of ChAdOx1 nCoV-19 Vaccine Administration in Thailand. *IJID Regions* 2. pp. 35–39. https://www.sciencedirect.com/science/article/pii/S2772707621000345.

First and foremost, it is important to note that the pre-pandemic state of the DMCs' health care systems was decisive in shaping outcomes and determining the kind of practices that were required in the first place. Pre-existing vaccine security efforts at the regional level or a fair global vaccination distribution system would have averted the need for aggressive diplomacy. Pre-existing high levels of credibility and trust (such as that enjoyed by Thailand's Ministry of Health) would have facilitated communications efforts. Similarly, the fact that Thailand and Viet Nam could pursue vaccine development as a "best practice" is contingent on having the infrastructure for such an initiative. As such, sustained investments in all of the areas mentioned above, as well as their enabling structural factors, is a necessary project that all countries can benefit from.

Second, as a matter of vaccine equity, there is a need to use a targeted approach that accounts for people's diverse geographic, demographic, socioeconomic, and cultural differences. In the highly populous Java-Bali area of Indonesia, for example, vaccinations were rolled out much faster in urban areas and noticeably slower in Outer Java-Bali and rural Indonesia (footnote 2). Targeted engagement should also consider specific age brackets. For instance, older people may not have much access to modern technology or a robust understanding of the science behind vaccines or young children, as identified by the Ministry of Health and City Center for Disease Control in Viet Nam, given the hesitancy among mothers to have their children vaccinated out of worries over side effects or assumptions that the children were supposedly too young to receive the vaccines. In these aspects, governments can work hand-in-hand with civil society organizations toward sustained local engagement with communities through discussions, health promotion, and outreach activities (footnote 15).

While the acute phase of the pandemic has passed, the medium- to long-term impacts of COVID-19 will doubtless continue to be felt. As such, countries must work toward developing stronger support for mental health services to frontline workers most impacted by the pandemic—in a manner of speaking, a "care for the carers" mechanism. At the same time, DMCs should also work on transitioning from providing COVID-19 vaccines via campaigns to integrating COVID-19 vaccination into routine immunization programs.[22] This will include maintaining or improving vaccination coverage levels, including those for present and future booster doses.

The advances in health- and vaccination-related technology must also be maintained. The case of Indonesia has demonstrated how crucial its One Data information management system has been to big-data capacity development in the country, allowing transparent, cross-sectoral review of governmental guidelines and their subsequent implementation. However, that system remains imperfect. It receives many different data sources from various subnational governments that have also developed their own information systems, but these sources need to be extracted and integrated into a national system. So far, this local-to-national data transfer system has put additional strain on an already resource-constrained setting, posing concerns about data quality. Moreover, apart from system interoperability amid the country's institutional and geographical fragmentation, there is also a lack of trained health human resources who can work on the system to

[22] G. Gotsadze et al. 2023. Adult Vaccination in Asia and the Pacific: Policies, Financial Needs, and Fiscal Impacts. *ADB Sustainable Development Working Paper Series* No. 90. ADB. https://www.adb.org/publications/adult-vaccination-asia-pacific.

preserve data quality and integrity (footnote 14). In the long run, better tracking and data-storage technologies will inevitably make vaccinations more efficient—and the identification of low-uptake areas easier for the government.

This is where partnerships between the government and the private sector can prove useful. A case study in Yogyakarta, Indonesia, for example, showed how One Data information has often been hampered by unstable access to the system and the untimely entry of data by workers who have other health-related tasks to deal with. Moving forward, the Government of Indonesia can leverage collaboration between the government and the private sector, not only for COVID-19 but for the health system as a whole.[23]

The Philippines has also shown how fruitful PPPs can be in improving health service delivery. In a country with a highly privatized health care system, the private sector can play a more involved role in developing new health care technologies and innovations. Investing in research and development to improve the quality and efficiency of health services and broadening the capacities of information technology in health.

[23] Partnership for Australia-Indonesia Centre. 2021. One Data: COVID-19, Health Data Connectivity and Integration in Indonesia–A Case Study of Yogyakarta. *The Australia-Indonesia Centre.* 4 August. https://pair.australiaindonesiacentre.org/featured/one-data-covid-19-health-data-connectivity-and-integration-in-indonesia-a-case-study-of-yogyakarta/.

CHAPTER 2

Communicating Vaccines and Countering Hesitancy

KEY POINTS

- Vaccine hesitancy—shaped by the three C's of credibility, complacency, and convenience—remains a significant barrier to successful immunization in the region.
- Communication and stakeholder engagement interventions must be (i) agile and evidence-based, (ii) low maintenance and replicable, and (iii) tailored and targeted.
- Following the three C's, countering hesitancy involves rebuilding and bolstering trust on health authorities, improving people's levels of risk perception toward COVID-19 and other infectious diseases, making vaccine-related services user-friendly, and creatively communicating all of the above to communities.

This chapter discusses vaccine hesitancy in Southeast Asia (i.e., the delay in acceptance or refusal of vaccines despite the availability of vaccine services).[24] It draws on insights from a regional stakeholder meeting in October 2022 and from the regional literature that has emerged since the start of the pandemic to identify best practices and offer recommendations for vaccine communications and stakeholder engagement. Aside from their applicability to the ongoing pandemic, these insights can prove useful to future pandemics, health crises, and general immunization programs in the region and elsewhere, given that vaccine-preventable diseases share the same challenges as COVID-19.

Even before the first COVID-19 vaccines were administered at the end of 2020, health communication experts had already anticipated the unique challenges this gargantuan effort would pose to public health authorities worldwide. For one, these were new vaccines being developed for a new disease, not to mention that multiple companies were manufacturing different types of vaccines. Second, their development, from the stages of clinical trials to public rollout, was much faster than any other vaccine, raising understandable public concerns over their safety and efficacy. Further complicating communications efforts was the difficulty of explaining to the public how and why certain groups were prioritized.

[24] Strategic Advisory Group of Experts (SAGE). 2014. *Report of the SAGE Working Group on Vaccine Hesitancy*. Compass. https://thecompassforsbc.org/sbcc-tools/report-sage-working-group-vaccine-hesitancy#:~:text=The%20SAGE%20Working%20Group%20on%20Vaccine%20Hesitancy%20developed%20a%20vaccine,not%20yet%20been%20psychometrically%20evaluated.

In identifying the challenges DMCs face in the region, this chapter uses the Strategic Advisory Group of Experts (SAGE) model as an analytic framework. This model identifies three determinants of vaccine hesitancy: confidence, complacency, and convenience. The first factor, confidence, calls attention to people's trust in the vaccines themselves, the health facilities and authorities delivering them, and the government mechanisms that enable the program (i.e., budget, procurement process). The second, complacency, refers to lowered risk perception when an individual does not see vaccination as imperative to disease prevention, or when the disease is no longer seen as a threat. Finally, convenience is "measured by the extent to which physical availability, affordability and willingness-to-pay, geographical accessibility, ability to understand (language and health literacy) and appeal of immunization services affect uptake (footnote 24)."

Vaccine Hesitancy in the Region

Before and during the initial vaccine rollouts, some surveys were conducted to gauge people's acceptance of the COVID-19 vaccines. At the time, some brands were still undergoing approval processes while others were already being administered. In four of the most populous countries in Southeast Asia (Indonesia, the Philippines, Thailand, and Viet Nam), the surveys yielded varying results. In Indonesia, a study jointly conducted by the Ministry of Health, UNICEF, and WHO found an initial acceptance rate of 64.8%, with only 8% of respondents saying they would refuse vaccination.[25] Those figures, however, differed from the findings of a study by an Indonesian research firm, which indicated that only 37% were willing to get the vaccines once they were available.[26] In the same vein, a few months after mass vaccinations started in the Philippines, surveys conducted by two independent research agencies each showed more than 50% hesitancy rate,[27] while the study conducted by the country's Department of Health revealed a relatively lower figure, around 25%.[28] In Thailand, a polling agency reported that more than 60% of its respondents expressed willingness to get vaccinated in the initial months of the rollout.[29] Available studies in Viet Nam were more recent and conducted by local and international institutions in 2022. They found a rate of just over 20% for vaccine hesitancy among the local population.[30]

The significant rates of vaccine hesitancy across the region, from the pre- and initial phases of the rollouts up to when boosters were already being offered, can be attributed to various factors.

---

25 UNICEF. 2020. *COVID-19 Vaccine Acceptance Survey in Indonesia.* https://www.unicef.org/indonesia/media/7631/file/COVID-19%20Vaccine%20Acceptance%20Survey%20in%20Indonesia.pdf.

26 Saiful Mujani Research & Consulting. 2020. *Kepercayaan Publik Nasional pada Vaksin dan Vaksinasi COVID-19.* https://saifulmujani.com/kepercayaan-publik-nasional-pada-vaksin-dan-vaksinasi-COVID-19/.

27 Mindanao Development Authority. 2021. *MinDa Survey*; and Pulse Asia. 2021. *Ulat ng Bayan Nationwide Survey*.

28 Government of the Philippines, Department of Health. 2021. *DOH COVID-19 Vaccine Survey*.

29 Suan Dusit University. 2021. *Suan Dusit Poll.*

30 R. R. Marzo et al. 2022. Hesitancy in COVID-19 Vaccine Uptake and Its Associated Factors among the General Adult Population: A Cross-Sectional Study in Six Southeast Asian Countries. *Tropical Medicine and Health.* 50 (4); and H. V. Nhu et al. 2022. COVID-19 Vaccine Acceptance in Viet Nam: An Online Cross-Sectional Study. *Asia Pacific Journal of Public Health.* 34 (1). pp. 131–133.

In the Ministry of Health-UNICEF-WHO study in Indonesia, the respondents identified distrust toward vaccine safety as the main reason for refusal (footnote 25). A survey in the Philippines similarly identified this factor as a top concern among the vaccine-hesitant, with 66% of people in 2021 claiming they were worried about experiencing side effects.[31] Similarly, the Thailand study showed that 59% of respondents were concerned about adverse events following immunization (AEFI) (footnote 29). In Viet Nam, a 2022 study found that those who were aware of the potential health complications vaccines could cause were less likely to get vaccinated.[32]

Distrust in the vaccines' effectiveness also played a role in people's low levels of confidence to get vaccinated. In the Philippines, the United Nations Development Programme (UNDP) highlighted the concerns about vaccine ineffectiveness as among the top reasons for hesitancy (footnote 31). More than a fifth of respondents in the Ministry of Health-UNICEF-WHO survey in Indonesia said the same thing (footnote 25), which was reaffirmed by another local study conducted in 2022.[33] In Thailand, social media users openly criticized the government's adoption of a mixed-vaccine protocol, questioning both the effectiveness and safety of administering doses as such.

Even among supposed key advocates of COVID-19 vaccination, there were reports of vaccine hesitancy, further underscoring the prevalence of this concern. A study among health workers in Thailand attributed hesitancy to perceived vaccine ineffectiveness and safety-related issues.[34] In Viet Nam, although 76.1% of health workers confirmed acceptance of the COVID-19 vaccines, one-fifth still said they were hesitant to receive them.[35]

Factors Behind Vaccine Hesitancy

Sociocultural and political factors were evident causes of hesitancy. A 2021 study in Indonesia's predominantly Muslim society found that more than 80% of those surveyed would accept the vaccines only if they were halal.[36] In the Philippines, religious concerns included the belief that the vaccines would "replace God's created natural antibodies."[37]

---

31 UNDP Philippines. 2021. *Trends in COVID-19 Vaccine Acceptance in the Philippines and Their Implications on Health Communication*. https://www.undp.org/philippines/publications/trends-covid-19-vaccine-acceptance-philippines-and-their-implications-health-communication.

32 H. V. Nhu et al. 2022. COVID-19 Vaccine Acceptance in Viet Nam: An Online Cross-Sectional Study. *Asia Pacific Journal of Public Health*. 34 (1). pp. 131–133.

33 A. Utami et al. 2022. Determinant Factors of COVID-19 Vaccine Hesitancy Among Adult and Elderly Population in Central Java, Indonesia. *Patient Preference and Adherence*. 16. pp. 1559–1570. https://doi.org/10.2147/PPA.S365663.

34 C. Pheerapanyawaranun et al. 2022. COVID-19 Vaccine Hesitancy among Health Care Workers in Thailand: The Comparative Results of Two Cross-Sectional Online Surveys before and after Vaccine Availability. *Frontiers in Public Health*. 10. 834545. https://doi.org/10.3389/fpubh.2022.834545.

35 G. Huynh et al. 2021. COVID-19 Vaccination Intention among Healthcare Workers in Viet Nam. *Asian Pacific Journal of Tropical Medicine*. 14 (4).pp. 159–164.

36 Indikator Politik Indonesia. 2021. *Siapa enggan Divaksin? Tantangan dan Problem Vaksinasi Covid-19 Di Indonesia*. https://indikator.co.id/wp-content/uploads/2021/02/Materi-Rilis-Indikator-Feb_21-02-2021.pdf.

37 A. M. L. Amit et al. 2022. COVID-19 Vaccine Brand Hesitancy and Other Challenges to Vaccination in the Philippines. *PLOS Glob Public Health*. 2 (1). pp. 1–23. https://journals.plos.org/globalpublichealth/article?id=10.1371/journal.pgph.0000165.

Another common narrative on the lack of trust in COVID-19 vaccines concerned the vaccines' origins, which companies manufactured them, and which countries they originated from. In the Philippines, research suggested that Filipinos' negative perception of vaccines from the People's Republic of China (PRC) could be related to political issues, including the territorial disputes between the two countries.[38] Many people expressed mistrust or distrust over the vaccines developed by companies from the PRC. Not only were these vaccines perceived as less effective than their Western counterparts, but the public also questioned the motivation of their respective governments in procuring them—a recurring narrative in social media conversations. Additionally, some people also felt they were only being "experimented on" by local and international authorities, given that the vaccines were already being offered to people despite the lack of full approval from the national regulatory authority (footnote 37).

Trust in COVID-19 vaccines and state-led vaccination programs might have also been influenced by a history of vaccine-related misinformation and controversies. For example, the issue of the vaccines' halal status in Indonesia was a narrative already pointed out by a 2019 study on measles vaccination coverage in the country.[39] A study in 2016 in Viet Nam found that 68.2% of its respondents would be hesitant to receive vaccines after hearing about AEFIs, while 12.4% would refuse vaccines if AEFIs had come up before.[40] In the Philippines, the 2016 rollout of a dengue vaccine that allegedly caused the death of more than 600 children, most of whom were infants,[41] and the subsequent, highly publicized hearings and trials of concerned government authorities and vaccine manufacturers have continued to haunt vaccination programs in the country (footnote 38).

Complacency has also been observed in the region. A 2021 study among older adults in Thailand found that the decreasing trend of COVID-19 cases contributed to people's complacency and consequently informed their attitude toward seeking vaccination.[42] Similarly, 45% of respondents in a study by the International Organization for Migration (IOM) in Thailand among Cambodian and Burmese migrant workers in the country expressed hesitancy by pointing out that vaccines were not necessary for "[already] healthy people."[43] In the Philippines, the same sentiment was raised by young participants of one study, where respondents mentioned that they could survive COVID-19 even without getting vaccinated (footnote 37).

---

38 R. J. Vergara. 2021. Social Trauma as a Contributory Factor in Filipino's Vaccine Hesitancy. *Journal of Public Health*. 43 (4). pp. e745–e746. https://doi.org/10.1093/pubmed/fdab110.

39 P. Pronyk et al. 2019. Vaccine Hesitancy in Indonesia. *The Lancet Planetary Health*. 3 (3). pp. E114–E115. https://doi.org/10.1016/S2542-5196(18)30287-0.

40 B. X. Tran et al. 2018. Media Representation of Vaccine Side Effects and Its Impact on Utilization of Vaccination Services in Viet Nam. *Patient Preference and Adherence*. 12. pp. 1717–1728.

41 C. Isoux. 2019. Are Philippine Children's Deaths Linked to Dengue Vaccine? *South China Morning Post*. 21 April. https://www.scmp.com/magazines/post-magazine/long-reads/article/3006712/philippines-suspicion-dengue-vaccine-linked.

42 Prachachat. 2021. *Vaccine hesitancy: bpà-dtì-sèt ráp vaccine · pai kúk-kaam tóp 10* [*Vaccine Hesitancy: Refusal to Vaccinate, Top 10 Threats*]. https://www.prachachat.net/general/news-794922.

43 IOM Thailand. 2022. https://displacement.iom.int/sites/g/files/tmzbdl1461/files/reports/COVID19_VaccinePerception_Jul26.pdf.

In terms of convenience, the distance of people's homes or workplaces to vaccination centers and the associated costs of getting from one place to another contributed to hesitancy in Viet Nam.[44] Likewise, a UNDP study in the Philippines found that one reason for not getting vaccinated was the time spent undergoing the process (actual versus expected time).[45] That study highlighted how many among the respondents with the lowest vaccine confidence theoretically had to travel for at least 1 hour from their residence to the designated vaccination sites, with the whole process predicted to take up to 3 hours (these respondents said they were willing to allot only 2 hours for the process).

Taken together, all these findings, which have been confirmed by more recent studies,[46] make it clear that all three determinants of vaccine hesitancy—credibility, complacency, convenience—must be addressed in Southeast Asian countries. Although there is a need for a more comprehensive and systematized regional study on vaccine hesitancy to collectively address the region's challenges, the existing data suggest that

(i) Serious concerns about vaccine safety, particularly on AEFIs, continue to negatively impact confidence in vaccines.
(ii) While low levels of complacency exist, this still needs to be sufficiently addressed as governments continue to ease or outright abolish pandemic-related restrictions. This will also be relevant in the face of the possibly waning effectiveness of existing vaccines against new COVID-19 virus subvariants.
(iii) Vaccine brand preference has significantly contributed to people's decisions to delay vaccinations.
(iv) More should be done to make the vaccines more accessible.

As countries move forward with the next phases of their COVID-19 vaccination campaigns and prepare for future ones, the question now becomes: How will health communications and stakeholder engagement contribute to addressing the challenges related to vaccination confidence, convenience, and complacency (Table 2)?

Table 2: Determinants of Vaccine Hesitancy

Factor	Regional Challenges	Best Practices
Credibility	Perceptions of mistrust toward national health authorities, the government, and vaccines (including specific vaccine brands)	Embarking on campaigns to counter disinformation, working with various sectors and local communities to build trust
Complacency	Decreasing morbidity, severity, and mortality, making people feel they do not need vaccines	Working with various sectors and local communities toward a "persuasive approach" using creativity in communicating risk
Convenience	Concerns about having to travel or spending too much time to get vaccinated	Making facilities more accessible and comfortable, making the vaccination process more efficient from appointment to receiving the shot

44 D. M. Duong et al. 2020. Controlling the COVID-19 Pandemic in Viet Nam: Lessons from a Limited Resource Country. *Asia Pacific Journal of Public Health*. 32 (4). pp. 161–162.

45 UNDP Philippines. 2021. Trends in COVID-19 Vaccine Acceptance in the Philippines and Their Implications on Health Communication. https://www.undp.org/philippines/publications/trends-covid-19-vaccine-acceptance-philippines-and-their-implications-health-communication.

46 Johns Hopkins Center for Communication Programs. (2022). COVID Behaviors Dashboard. https://ccp.jhu.edu/kap-covid/.

Addressing Vaccine Hesitancy Through Communications and Stakeholder Engagement

A common misconception is that communication activities alone can counter vaccine hesitancy. Indeed, in the words of SAGE, "communication remains a critical tool to manage vaccine hesitancy. It cannot only improve knowledge, influence policy, the environment, and realize behavioral changes (footnote 24)." As WHO's SAGE and other public health bodies have emphasized, communication is one of many tools at the disposal of the public health system(footnote 24). Mindful of this, the following points can be drawn from regional experience and serve as starting points for conceptualizing ways forward:

(i) Strong pandemic leadership—characterized, among others, by having "one voice" from the authorities—promotes trust. That is to say, "trust springs from credibility."[47] As the main currency of communications during public health emergencies, trust is important not only between the public and their leaders but also between the public and scientific bodies in charge of generating pandemic-related knowledge and data. As Thailand's experience shows, communication was key to its pandemic response, even as pandemic outcomes also help determine the government's credibility in the eyes of the people.[48]

(ii) Collaboration with the media, development partners, the academe, the private sector, and entire communities is critical during emergencies, but systems and mechanisms to engage them must be strengthened or institutionalized. This is because responses and communication efforts should not be one-sided; they have to be participatory (footnote 47). For instance, the involvement of youth leaders helped tailor a "persuasive approach" to vaccination in parts of Indonesia.

(iii) Much work remains to be done in terms of infodemic management. This includes, among others: (a) widening our understanding of infodemic management, which should go beyond countering misinformation and disinformation on social media; (b) improving access to relevant and affordable tools for knowledge sharing; and (c) systematizing mechanisms to manage infodemics.[49] Toward this end, the collation and analysis of the experiences of various ministries of health (as well as other government agencies) in countering misinformation during COVID-19 using social media and other tools would be an invaluable resource.

(iv) Evidence and data are key to contextualized communication responses. Thus, there should be more investment in the swift generation of scientific evidence for practical guidance, particularly on risk perception and behavioral insights. In the Philippines, specialty societies came up with "living recommendations" to interpret "rapidly evolving science",[50] an initiative that can inspire similar efforts from social science and communications bodies and strengthened with official support and greater collaboration with academic institutions.

---

[47] G. Lasco and V. G. Yu. 2021. Communicating COVID-19 Vaccines: Lessons from the Dengue Vaccine Controversy in the Philippines. *BMJ Global Health* 6. e005422.

[48] P. Slutskiy and S. Boonchutima. 2022. Credibility of the Official COVID Communication in Thailand: When People Stop Believing the Government. *American Behavioral Scientist*. 00027642221118297.

[49] L. P. Wong et al. 2020. Vaccine Hesitancy and the Resurgence of Vaccine Preventable Diseases: The Way Forward for Malaysia, a Southeast Asian Country. *Human Vaccines & Immunotherapeutics*. 16 (7). pp. 1511–1520.

[50] Philippine Society for Microbiology and Infectious Diseases. 2023. Philippine COVID-19 Living Recommendations. 27 June. https://www.psmid.org/philippine-covid-19-living-recommendations-3/.

(v) There is a need for quicker mechanisms for countries and institutions to share their success stories for contextualized application.
(vi) Committed leadership from governments must be translated into action and concrete results. If no commitment has been made, stronger advocacy is necessary to ensure that health communication capacities are systematized and rendered sustainable.

Building on these overarching lessons, three characteristics of health communication and stakeholder engagement interventions can guide countries in the region moving forward: (i) agile and evidence-based, (ii) low maintenance and replicable, and (iii) tailored and targeted.

Agile and Evidence-Based

Responses to disease outbreaks and other public health emergencies should be fast-paced. This has held true for COVID-19 and newly developed vaccines. Since the first rollouts, there have been many changes to the virus and the vaccines, which has meant that new information needs to be communicated to the public in the most appropriate yet cost-effective channels.

Agility is the ability to improve performance amid challenges and regardless of disruptions and to be able to learn and grow from them.[51] It entails not only speed but also flexibility and creativity to ensure that interventions continue to address the present challenges despite sudden changes and with minimal but significant adjustments.

Speed is a determinant of agility. In health communications, however, ensuring that an activity is evidence-based can be seen as a hindrance to speeding up. However, there should not be a tradeoff between these two factors. Because evidence generation is generally viewed as a resource-intensive task, more investment is necessary to improve capabilities to conduct it more efficiently.

Low Maintenance and Replicable

Having the necessary temporal, financial, and human resources is critical to sustaining potentially effective interventions. This holds true, especially for emergency responses where the authorities' workload increases significantly. Unfortunately, resources allotted for health communication have remained limited in many countries, as this area of work is still largely viewed as an ad hoc activity. Funding is insufficient, relevant units and departments are not adequately staffed, and in some cases, health communications is merely an extra task assigned to health workers with other priorities.

Of course, the best-case scenario is that health communications is made a priority. Given unfavorable realities in many countries, however, practitioners must ensure that all interventions are planned in the least resource-intensive way. What matters most is that interventions fulfill their purpose and are sustainable.

[51] M. Wade et al. 2021. 6 Principles to Build Your Company's Strategic Agility. *Harvard Business Review*. 2 September. https://hbr.org/2021/09/6-principles-to-build-your-companys-strategic-agility.

If health communication and stakeholder engagement interventions were low maintenance, they would also be easier to replicate not only from national to subnational levels but also from one country to another. During the COVID-19 pandemic, knowledge and experience sharing across countries has become a key component of global solidarity. Countries have been sharing how they successfully implemented their respective, effective measures and interventions, including in health communication, for others to potentially implement as well.

Tailored and Targeted

Mass communication strategies (e.g., the use of mass media and mass public relations campaigns) can feel like a convenient way to reach entire populations. However, a "one-size-fits-all" approach is not always applicable across populations, groups, and individuals. Socioeconomic contexts, geographic factors, and cultural values shape people's decision-making processes. Thus, when health authorities communicate, they should aim for the change they want to see among the people they are talking to. In the case of COVID-19 vaccinations, this has meant recognizing that some populations, like older adults or migrant workers, would have required more tailored and targeted approaches because of their different contexts. For example, "a moratorium on the prosecution of undocumented migrants" could have encouraged uptake among a country's migrant population at a time when all individuals, regardless of legal status, must have ideally been vaccinated.[52]

Recommendations

As the world moves past the pandemic, the challenge for public health authorities remains threefold, mirroring WHO's SAGE framework but likewise drawing from regional lessons learned:

(i) Increase people's confidence in vaccines in general by (re)building and bolstering trust in the authorities administering them, the mechanisms being used and, of course, the vaccines themselves.
(ii) Decrease people's complacency by raising their levels of risk perception toward COVID-19 and appropriately managing similar perceptions for other infectious diseases.
(iii) Improve convenience of accessing vaccine-related services and creatively communicate such convenience to communities.

To achieve these, future health communication and stakeholder engagement interventions must be agile and evidence-based, low maintenance and replicable, and tailored and targeted (ALT). Based on these principles, here are key tasks for the near future.

52 Y. Teerawattananon et al. 2021. Vaccinating Undocumented Migrants against Covid-19. *BMJ* 373. n1608. https://doi.org/10.1136/bmj.n1608.

Identify and Map Stakeholders and Continue Harnessing Partnerships with Them

COVID-19 has shown that while subject matter expertise is important in gaining and maintaining people's trust, proximity, track record, and established relationships, it also plays a critical role in convincing people that the vaccines being offered to them are safe and effective. Early identification of stakeholders, as well as mapping them according to the support they could potentially provide, will be vital for future vaccination rollouts.

A single report on national television can make or break a vaccination campaign—media partners are that powerful. Civil society, community-based, and religious organizations have well-established relationships with entire communities that can be easily tapped when encouraging people to get vaccinated. Some development partners, including international organizations, also have a wide reach through their respective platforms and channels that can be used for quick communications and countering vaccine-related misinformation. Celebrities, social media influencers, and other key opinion leaders have significant numbers of followers who listen to and are influenced by them. Health workers, especially those at primary care facilities, have direct, regular interactions with their patients and remain among the public's most trusted sources of health information. Having one voice with these stakeholders and being on the same page with them in terms of vaccine-related messaging can increase the public's trust in vaccines and vaccination programs.

Partnerships can also effectively improve and communicate vaccine accessibility. Non-state actors, including the private sector and academe, had massive resources to offer throughout the course of vaccination campaigns in the past 3 years. These included providing transportation and other logistical assistance to bring vaccines to remote communities, improving vaccination scheduling systems, lending huge venues for mass vaccination drives, and employing their own means of commercial marketing to communicate vaccines to the people.

These partnerships should be maintained in the subsequent phases of COVID-19 vaccination campaigns. The "last mile" in many countries involves remote communities, and the logistical support these partners can offer will significantly help bring the vaccines closer to people. Commercial marketing techniques employed by companies to sell products and services can also be effective in clearly communicating the procedures for vaccination early on, thereby managing people's expectations as they undergo these procedures. These techniques can potentially supplement the likely limited-resourced communication strategies to be implemented by public health authorities.

Where the above collaborations do not exist yet, governments should endeavor to identify potential partners, connect with them, and create formal mechanisms to start working with them.

Establish an Intersectoral Task Force for Vaccine Communication

After potential stakeholders have been identified and mapped, they should be systematically engaged in crafting the subsequent phases of vaccine communication strategies. One way to do this is to establish an institutional body, such as an intersectoral task force or steering committee composed of government authorities, partners, and other stakeholders. Such a mechanism worked well during the various phases of many countries' COVID-19 responses and would be critical for the next phases of vaccination campaigns. The task force's responsibilities may include:

(i) prioritizing strategies for execution, especially regarding vaccination of the "last mile";
(ii) communicating policy updates from the national technical advisory group on immunization;
(iii) managing crisis communication response, such as during AEFI;
(iv) maintaining and updating an online database and repository of materials that may be useful for the next phase of the vaccination campaigns;
(v) building local capacity to periodically assess and respond to communication needs; and
(vi) building knowledge by allocating funds for formative research and impact evaluation to ensure that the planned interventions will be contextualized and evidence-based.

Systematize Mechanisms for Combating Misinformation

COVID-19 vaccines have been hugely victimized by misinformation, negatively impacting people's confidence in them. At the national and subnational levels, the task of fighting misinformation has been carried out mainly through the support of external partners or in an ad hoc, unsystematic manner. Sustaining efforts around this area have been unsuccessful in many countries, especially after their respective COVID-19 situations became relatively controlled.

Certain country experiences of the pandemic have highlighted the importance of investing in systematic mechanisms that challenge misinformation in this age of social media. For example, Indonesia launched a nationwide misinformation awareness campaign in 2021 by having government and private sector actors working collectively across traditional and social media platforms within a specific, immediate time frame.[53] Having the right tools and expertise in place, and financing them sustainably is critical not only to fulfill the remaining COVID-19 vaccination targets but also to protect future vaccination campaigns for other diseases.

Communicate More Creatively with Target Audiences

In many cases, simply telling people the facts, even through easily understandable language, will not really convince them to follow the recommended actions (e.g., making them read communication materials written in plain language). Up to now, many countries have continued to struggle with persuading portions of their population to get their COVID-19 booster doses, given the decreasing number of COVID-19 cases and the recession of the pandemic in the public consciousness.

Persuasion is important in health communication because it ensures that the target audiences do not blindly follow authorities. When persuaded, they take action because they are convinced it is the right thing to do. The presence of logos, ethos, and pathos is critical in persuasion. Logos appeals to an individual's reason—why one should agree with the message being sent. Ethos appeals to an individual's perception of authority—why one should trust

[53] R. Triwardani. 2021. Indonesian Officials and Media Fight Vaccine Hesitancy, Misinformation. *Asia Politics & Policy*. 13 (4). pp. 635–639. 10.1111/.aspp.12608.

the bearer of the message. Lastly, pathos appeals to an individual's emotions, which makes it possible for target audiences to relate to the message. Combining all three in health communications requires the authorities to understand their target audiences' socioeconomic and cultural contexts, as well as family and community dynamics, among other factors.

Thus, health communications have to be delivered more creatively and innovatively to reach as many people as possible in the most efficient way possible. One possible method, as mentioned earlier, is getting social media influencers to participate in informational campaigns, especially in countries like the Philippines with high rates of social media usage;[54] in fact, this method was used in Indonesia, where influencers were considered a priority group in the early months of vaccinations.[55]

---

54 E. Bonnevie et al. 2021. Social Media Influencers Can Be Used to Deliver Positive Information About the Flu Vaccine: Findings from a Multi-Year Study. *Health Education Research*. 36 (3). pp. 286–294. https://doi.org/10.1093/her/cyab018.

55 S. Widianto and K. Lamb. 2021. Instagram Influencers Are a Vaccine Priority in Wary Indonesia. *Reuters*. 14 January. https://www.reuters.com/business/media-telecom/instagram-influencers-are-vaccine-priority-wary-indonesia-2021-01-14/.

CHAPTER 3

Digitizing Vaccine Information Systems

KEY POINTS

- Vaccine information systems (VISs) have played a critical role in the distribution, administration, and monitoring of COVID-19 vaccines in the region.
- The success of VIS depended on structural factors including levels of literacy, geography, and digital infrastructure.
- Regional experience underscores the need to invest in widely accessible, user-friendly, interoperable, and secure digital infrastructure; promote stakeholder engagement, address vaccine hesitancy; ensure standardization; and encourage a regional surveillance system.
- If sustained, these systems can enable and strengthen health security in the region.

A vaccine information system (VIS) is an electronic system used to collect, manage, and apply immunization data to support vaccination programs. Since the 1990s, it has been recognized as having the potential to greatly improve the planning, implementation, and evaluation of vaccination programs by providing timely and accurate data.[56] VISs can help identify vaccine-preventable diseases and populations at risk and monitor vaccine coverage and adverse events following immunization. As such, a VIS is a critical component of any vaccination program, as it provides comprehensive and up-to-date records of individuals who have received vaccinations, allowing for the monitoring of vaccine safety and efficacy and enabling the timely identification of outbreaks or clusters of vaccine-preventable diseases.

Within Southeast Asia, immunization efforts have been pivotal in preventing millions of deaths and disabilities, leading to the establishment of robust immunization systems and substantial reductions in morbidities and mortalities from once highly endemic diseases. In early 2014, for example, the WHO Southeast Asia Region became the fourth WHO

[56] D. Wood et al. 1999. Immunization registries in the United States: implications for the practice of public health in a changing health care system. *Annual Review of Public Health*. 20 (1). pp. 231–255. doi:10.1146/annurev.publhealth.20.1.231.

region to receive polio-free certification, underscoring the region's successful efforts in controlling and eradicating this devastating disease. VISs have been central to these disease prevention and immunization-related efforts by making vaccination programs more efficient and effective in providing accurate and timely information on vaccine demand, supply, and coverage.

In the context of the COVID-19 pandemic, VISs played a critical role in the distribution, administration, and monitoring of COVID-19 vaccines in many parts of the world, including several countries in Southeast Asia. While some countries, most notably Viet Nam, had already implemented a VIS before COVID-19, it was only during the pandemic that efforts to develop such systems were accelerated in many other places.[57] Even so, certain challenges have persisted, including the equitable distribution of vaccines across geographically diverse regions, disparities in logistics and health care infrastructure, and the need for sustainable financing to procure vaccines and essential equipment.

To better understand the strengths and weaknesses of these VISs, this chapter draws on a scoping review to focus on five developing member countries (DMCs: Cambodia, Indonesia, the Philippines, Thailand, and Viet Nam), which were chosen based on their population size, diversity, and the different strategies implemented in response to the pandemic.[58] The chapter maps the literature on the VIS used in each country's COVID-19 response using the Preferred Reporting Items for Systematic Reviews and Meta-Analyses extension for scoping reviews. It explores the types of VIS used, their functionality, the challenges encountered, and lessons learned from their implementation. It then highlights the strengths and weaknesses of each country's VIS and its contributions to the COVID-19 response.

In so doing, this review can contribute to the body of knowledge on the use of VIS during the COVID-19 pandemic, particularly in Southeast Asia. Besides providing an overview of the status of VIS in each country, it also identifies the gaps in their implementation. This review concludes by providing recommendations related to post-COVID-19 and health security

---

[57] N. T. Nguyen et al. 2017. Digital Immunization Registry: Evidence for the Impact of mHealth on Enhancing the Immunization System and Improving Immunization Coverage for Children under One Year Old in Viet Nam. *mHealth* Vol. 3. https://mhealth.amegroups.com/article/view/15655/15718.

[58] This review was guided by the Preferred Reporting Items for Systematic Reviews and Meta-Analyses extension for scoping reviews and included articles published from December 2019 (when the first case of COVID-19 was reported in Wuhan, PRC) to March 2022. The exclusion criteria were as follows: (i) articles not conducted in Southeast Asia, (ii) not focused on VIS in each country's COVID-19 response, (iii) not published in English, and (iv) not peer-reviewed. Full-text articles were reviewed based on the same inclusion and exclusion criteria. Additionally, the review excluded grey literature such as reports, blogs, and opinion pieces. The search strategy aimed to identify studies related to VIS in Southeast Asia and each country's COVID-19 response. Five electronic databases were used to search for articles: PubMed, Scopus, Web of Science, Cochrane Library, and CINAHL. The following keywords and their combinations were used: "vaccine information system," "COVID-19," "Southeast Asia," "Philippines," "Indonesia," "Viet Nam," "Cambodia," and "Thailand." This search strategy was adapted for each database to match the specific syntax and keywords used. The initial search identified 531 articles, of which 77 were duplicates and subsequently removed. The remaining 454 articles were screened based on the inclusion and exclusion criteria, resulting in 23 articles that met the criteria for inclusion. The included studies were conducted from 2020 to 2022, with nine from the Philippines, six from Indonesia, four from Viet Nam, two from Cambodia, and two from Thailand. The study designs included 13 cross-sectional studies, seven qualitative studies, two case studies, and one mixed-methods study. The sample sizes ranged from 5 to 3,615 participants.

interventions drawn from the lessons learned from the implementation of VIS in Southeast Asia. These recommendations focus on the following areas: improving the functionality of VIS, enhancing the capacity of health systems to manage vaccination programs, ensuring equitable distribution of vaccines, addressing vaccine hesitancy, and strengthening health security systems.

Vaccine Information Systems by Country

VISs are essential tools in public health that facilitate the management, monitoring, and evaluation of vaccine administration. In Southeast Asia, VISs have been implemented in various forms, ranging from paper-based records to digital systems. The role of VISs has become increasingly crucial to the COVID-19 response as countries strive to vaccinate their populations to control the spread of the virus.

The implementation of VISs in Southeast Asia has been influenced by various factors, including the level of technological infrastructure, the availability of funding, and the regulatory framework governing vaccine administration. Countries in Southeast Asia have also adopted different approaches to implementing VIS, with some countries focusing on centralized systems and others prioritizing decentralized models.

Conclusions and Recommendations

This review has identified several challenges encountered in implementing VIS in each country's COVID-19 response. These challenges include inadequate digital infrastructure, limited resources, vaccine hesitancy, and low health literacy among the population.
In some countries, the lack of interoperability between different health information systems has been a challenge. Several lessons can also be gleaned from the implementation of VIS in each country. These include the importance of stakeholder engagement and collaboration, the need for adequate training and capacity building, the value of real-time data monitoring, and the importance of ensuring data privacy and security.

One of the limitations of this scoping review is the paucity of studies included in the analysis. Only 12 studies were identified for inclusion, which may not provide a comprehensive overview of the VIS used in each country's COVID-19 response. Additionally, the studies included in the review were mainly descriptive, and there were limited studies that evaluated the effectiveness of VIS in improving vaccination coverage or reducing the transmission of COVID-19. Furthermore, by only including studies published until March 2022, the review implicitly omits insights from more recent publications, given the evolving nature of the pandemic and countries' responses to it.

Nonetheless, this review has provided an adequate overview of the VIS used in each DMC's COVID-19 response. It has identified various types of VIS used, including web-based platforms, mobile applications, and digital health cards. While the functionalities of the VIS varied, most have been used to manage vaccine distribution, track the number of vaccinated individuals, and generate vaccination reports.

It is crucial to sustain the momentum of VIS implementation to improve health security and emergency preparedness. Based on this review, here are recommendations that could be made to enhance VIS in Southeast Asia.

Invest in Widely Accessible, User-Friendly, Interoperable, and Secure Digital Infrastructure

To ensure the successful implementation of VISs and other digital health interventions, countries should invest in digital infrastructure. Governments should prioritize investing in technology and digital literacy to promote the adoption of VIS and other digital health interventions. Strengthening the integration of VIS with other health information systems, such as disease surveillance and electronic health records, is critical to facilitating data sharing and improving health outcomes. This would also entail integrating the VIS into the existing health information systems to ensure interoperability. Finally, there is a need to ensure the sustainability of the systems beyond the COVID-19 response and to invest in the development of a robust regulatory framework to ensure the privacy and security of vaccine information data.

Collaborate and Engage with Stakeholders

The successful implementation of VIS requires collaboration among different stakeholders, including the government, health care providers, and community leaders. Governments should engage stakeholders and promote collaboration to facilitate the adoption of VIS and address the specific challenges encountered in each country. Beyond the literature on VISs, regional experience on digital health more broadly can be leveraged in pursuing this effort.[59]

Address Vaccine Hesitancy

Vaccine hesitancy is a significant challenge to the successful implementation of VIS. Governments should invest in communication campaigns that provide accurate information about the vaccines and combat misinformation. They should also collaborate with health care providers and community leaders to promote vaccine uptake and address vaccine hesitancy.

Develop a Standardized Vaccination Information System

To enable efficient monitoring of the vaccination program and facilitate cross-border travel, a standardized VIS across the region must be developed. The system should include unique QR codes that can be used to access vaccination records and monitor vaccine distribution and administration.

[59] For example, ADB. 2018. *Transforming Health Systems through Good Digital Health Governance*; ADB. 2018. *Digital Health Convergence Meeting Tool Kit*.

Establish a Regional Surveillance System

Establishing a regional surveillance system that can monitor disease outbreaks and vaccine-preventable diseases will help improve the region's health security. The system should be based on a standardized reporting system that enables real-time monitoring of disease outbreaks and vaccine-preventable diseases.

Overall, this review has highlighted the importance of VISs in supporting the COVID-19 response in Southeast Asia. It has also underscored the need for continued investment in these systems to strengthen health security and emergency preparedness in the region.

Cambodia

The VIS used were the Cambodian COVID-19 Vaccination Card and the Smart Green Hospital Network project. The Cambodian COVID-19 Vaccination Card is a digital health card that provides individuals with a unique identification number linked to their health records. The card contains personal health information, including medical history, allergies, and vaccination records. It is designed to facilitate access to health services, streamline patient identification, and support the efficient delivery of health care. In so doing, it enables accurate identification of individuals, ensuring they receive appropriate and timely health services. It also promotes continuity of care by providing health care providers access to comprehensive patient information, allowing informed decision-making and personalized care delivery.

On the other hand, the Smart Green Hospital Network is an electronic health record system that digitizes and centralizes patient health records. The system allows health care providers to securely access and update patient information, track medical histories, and facilitate seamless coordination of care across different facilities. It aims to improve health care delivery, enhance patient safety, and enable better decision-making by health care professionals by managing vaccine distribution and tracking the number of vaccinated individuals. The project enhances the quality and safety of health care services by centralizing patient records, reducing errors associated with paper-based systems, facilitating data sharing among health care providers, and improving coordination and continuity of care.

Additionally, the Cambodia Ministry of Health developed a web-based platform called the COVID-19 Vaccine Registration System (CVRS). The CVRS enables individuals to register for vaccination and provides them with a unique QR code that they can use to access their vaccination record. The system enables eligible individuals to register for vaccination, provides them with appointment details, and tracks vaccination progress. Thus, it helps streamline the vaccination process, ensures efficient allocation of vaccine doses, and enables timely communication with individuals regarding their vaccination status. Consequently, it supports data-driven decision-making, ensuring equitable vaccine distribution and coverage.

Cambodia's vaccination program has faced challenges such as supply shortages, logistical constraints, low health literacy, and vaccine hesitancy. To address these challenges, the government increased its vaccine procurement, launched a public information campaign to promote vaccine acceptance, and established a vaccine tracking system to monitor vaccine distribution. The government also collaborated with local authorities to conduct door-to-door campaigns to promote vaccine uptake.

Cambodia's implementation of the COVID-19 Vaccination Card, Smart Green Hospital Network project, and CVRS offers valuable lessons for other countries in the region. Firstly, integrating vaccination data into existing health information systems enhances data accuracy, accessibility, and efficiency. This integration enables a comprehensive view of an individual's health records, including vaccination history, facilitating targeted interventions and personalized health care. Countries should prioritize interoperability and integration to maximize the potential of their health information systems.

Digital platforms such as CVRS also streamline the vaccine registration process and ensure efficient vaccine distribution. Online registration systems reduce the burden on health care facilities, minimize long waiting times, and provide a convenient and accessible avenue for individuals to register for vaccination. Countries should explore similar digital solutions to optimize vaccine rollout and make access to vaccines more equitable.

To address vaccine hesitancy, Cambodia's VIS emphasized the importance of effective communication and community engagement. Public awareness campaigns, community outreach programs, and disseminating accurate vaccine information have played a significant role in building trust and addressing hesitancy. Countries should invest in comprehensive communication strategies, leveraging multiple channels to reach diverse populations. Engaging community leaders, influencers, and health care professionals as trusted sources of information can further enhance vaccine acceptance and uptake.

Indonesia

The information systems used were the Electronic Health Record system and the Sehati app. The system is a web-based platform that collects and manages health data. This was used to monitor vaccine inventory, track the number of vaccinated individuals, and generate vaccination reports. On the other hand, the Sehati app is used to schedule vaccination appointments and provide vaccination reminders. It offers various features such as telemedicine consultations, health records management, health education resources, and COVID-19 information. It is available in multiple languages and has a user-friendly interface that makes it accessible to a wide range of users, addressing potential language and digital literacy barriers. Through the app, users can access medical professionals, schedule appointments, and receive virtual care. At the height of the pandemic, the Sehati app aimed to enhance access to health care services by reducing the need for in-person visits and ensuring timely medical support. By facilitating remote consultations and providing essential health information, the app helped reduce the burden on health care facilities and enabled individuals to receive timely medical advice, ensuring that people could seek necessary care without physical contact.

Meanwhile, the COVID-19 Vaccination One Data System and PeduliLindungi app are two interconnected digital platforms used in Indonesia's COVID-19 response. The COVID-19 Vaccination One Data System serves as a central data repository, consolidating information related to COVID-19 cases, testing, vaccination, and health care facility capacities. The PeduliLindungi app, integrated with the One Data System, provides users with COVID-19 risk assessment, contact tracing, and health facility information. It also supports the issuance of digital vaccination certificates. Together, the two platforms demonstrate Indonesia's commitment to leveraging digital technologies for effective COVID-19 response, making vaccine distribution more equitable and contact tracing more efficient.

As part of the country's National Vaccination Program, the Indonesian Ministry of Health also implemented a digital platform called the Electronic Health Alert Card (eHAC) to register vaccine recipients, schedule appointments, and monitor vaccine distribution. Throughout the pandemic, the eHAC has served as a digital health pass system to monitor people's health status and travel history. The eHAC also collects information such as vaccination status, recent COVID-19 test results, and travel history, serving as a tool for authorities to track and manage potential health risks associated with travel. It is mandatory for domestic and international travelers to register on the eHAC platform before entering certain areas or boarding flights. Moreover, the eHAC enables individuals to register for vaccination and provides them with a unique QR code that they can use to access their vaccination records. In this way, it enables the monitoring of vaccine distribution and administration, as well as the generation of vaccination reports.

Indonesia's national program has faced challenges such as vaccine hesitancy, supply chain disruptions, and data quality issues. To address these challenges, the government has launched a public information campaign to promote vaccine acceptance and established a vaccine tracking system to monitor vaccine distribution. The Government of Indonesia has also collaborated with private companies and nongovernment organizations to establish vaccination centers and provide logistics support.

In terms of the supply (cold) chain system, Indonesia uses the SMILE app, which focuses on ensuring the integrity of vaccine distribution in Indonesia. The system monitors the temperature and condition of vaccines during storage and transportation. It uses real-time data, automated alerts, and temperature tracking devices to maintain the cold chain, ensuring that vaccines are stored and transported within the recommended temperature range. Thus, the system minimizes the risk of vaccine wastage and ensures that vaccines reach their intended recipients with their potency intact. Throughout the pandemic, this system has been crucial to effective vaccine distribution, especially for vaccines requiring specific temperature conditions.

Lastly, in terms of medical waste handling, the country uses SIKELIM (Sistem Informasi Kelola Limbah Medis). This information management system monitors medical waste generated during the COVID-19 response by tracking its collection, transportation, and disposal from health care facilities. The system ensures that medical waste is appropriately handled, treated, and disposed of in compliance with safety and environmental regulations. It thus minimizes the risk of environmental contamination and public health hazards, contributing to maintaining a safe and healthy environment for health care workers, patients, and the general population.

As in the Philippines, the Indonesian example points to the importance of elements like system integration and interoperability, user-centric design, and public awareness and engagement. Ensuring interoperability between different platforms allowed data to be shared across various stakeholders, enabling comprehensive monitoring and evaluation of the vaccination program's effectiveness. The user-centric design principles, such as intuitive navigation, multilingual support, and accessibility features, also helped promote inclusivity and facilitate equitable access to vaccination information. Moreover, to address vaccine hesitancy, the country also implemented a comprehensive public awareness campaign through PeduliLindungi, focusing on providing accurate information about COVID-19 vaccines, addressing common concerns, and dispelling misinformation.

Meanwhile, SMILE enabled end-to-end visibility of the vaccine cold chain, from manufacturing to administration. Beyond facilitating real-time monitoring of the cold chain, it optimized cold chain logistics through predictive analytics. Such analyses on vaccine demand, storage capacities, and transportation networks helped decision-makers plan vaccine distribution and address potential bottlenecks proactively. In terms of capacity building, implementing the cold supply chain system necessitated comprehensive training of health care workers and supply chain personnel, which meant that participants acquired the necessary skills to operate and manage the digital system effectively.

Lastly, SIKELIM has been instrumental in managing the disposal of medical waste generated during the COVID-19 vaccination campaign in Indonesia. On the one hand, it has streamlined medical waste management by digitizing documentation and improving traceability, ensuring better compliance with safety and environmental regulations. On the other hand, its real-time monitoring capabilities have enabled authorities to promptly identify any irregularities or deviations in medical waste management practices, ensuring immediate interventions to address potential risks such as improper waste handling. Collectively, the data in SIKELIM can be leveraged for informed decision-making and resource allocation. By analyzing trends and patterns in medical waste generation, decision-makers can identify areas of improvement, allocate resources more effectively, and implement targeted interventions to enhance waste management practices.

Philippines

The DOH developed an online registration system called the COVID-19 Vaccine Information Management System (VIMS) in 2021. VIMS serves as a comprehensive information system that facilitates the registration, scheduling, and tracking of COVID-19 vaccine administration. It enables health care providers to record and manage vaccine recipients' data, including personal information, vaccination history, and adverse events. It also allows individuals to register for vaccination and provides them with a unique QR code that they can use to access their vaccination records. Moreover, VIMS enables the monitoring of vaccine distribution and administration, the generation of vaccination reports, and the provision of real-time data on vaccine inventory and utilization to inform decision-making.

A critical component of VIMS is VaxCertPH, which serves as a digital vaccine certificate or passport that provides individuals with proof of COVID-19 vaccination. The system generates a unique QR code linked to the individual's vaccination status, which can be easily verified by authorized personnel or establishments through a mobile app. VaxCertPH facilitates safe mobility, allowing individuals to present their digital vaccine certificate instead of physical documents when accessing certain venues or traveling. It has streamlined the verification process of individuals' vaccination status, offering a secure and convenient way to prove immunization. Digital vaccine certificates like this reduce the risk of fraud and enhance the efficiency of verification procedures—in effect, supporting the government's efforts to reopen the economy while ensuring public health safety by implementing stricter vaccination requirements in establishments.

Overall, implementing effective vaccine information systems, including the VIMS and VaxCertPH, contributed to the efficient and centralized management of the country's COVID-19 vaccination program, strengthening health security, ensuring equitable vaccine distribution, and addressing vaccine hesitancy. It has improved data accuracy, accessibility, and reporting capabilities, allowing policymakers and health authorities to make informed decisions based on real-time information. The system's ability to track and monitor vaccination coverage has helped identify areas with low immunization rates, enabling targeted interventions to ensure equitable vaccine distribution.

One of the key lessons learned from implementing VIMS is the importance of seamless integration with existing health information systems. By ensuring interoperability, VIMS can exchange data with other platforms, such as electronic health records and surveillance systems. This integration enhances data accuracy, minimizes duplication, and facilitates a comprehensive understanding of the vaccination landscape.

The success of the VaxCertPH was primarily driven by its user-friendly interface and strict privacy safeguards. It is essential to ensure that individuals can easily access their vaccination records while protecting their personal information. Clear communication about data privacy measures, informed consent, and transparent governance frameworks help build trust in the system and encourage widespread adoption.

Another lesson, particularly for a geographically diverse country like the Philippines, is the importance of broad access to digital infrastructure and ensuring the capacity of human workers to use the system or, if needed, to offer alternative solutions. In areas with difficult or no internet access, the DOH had to set up on-site vaccination sites for people to schedule appointments and resorted to the more widely available text messaging.

The experience of the Philippines with vaccine information systems, exemplified by VIMS and VaxCertPH, offers valuable insights and best practices for strengthening health security and promoting equitable vaccine distribution. The integration of these systems, along with a focus on interoperability, user accessibility, privacy protection, and targeted public awareness campaigns, has contributed to the successful management of the vaccination process and the mitigation of vaccine hesitancy.

Thailand

The VIS used was the Mor Prom (or Doctors Ready) platform. It was developed by the Government of Thailand to streamline and facilitate the vaccination process. The platform served as a comprehensive solution to vaccine registration, appointment scheduling, and vaccination monitoring. It ensured efficient vaccine distribution, enhanced data management, and enabled effective communication between health care providers and vaccine recipients. It also allowed health care providers to track vaccine distribution, monitor vaccination coverage, and manage inventory effectively. Real-time data on vaccine availability and utilization can help identify areas that require additional resources or targeted interventions, ensuring equitable distribution of vaccines across the country.

The Mor Prom app allows individuals to register for vaccination and provides them with a unique QR code that they can use to access their vaccination records. It also enables the monitoring of vaccine distribution and administration and the generation of vaccination reports. Moreover, the platform allows individuals to register for COVID-19 vaccination through various channels, including a mobile application, website, or designated registration centers. Once registered, individuals receive confirmation and are provided with an appointment date and time for their vaccination. The platform also supports health care providers by providing them with real-time information on vaccine availability, scheduling, and inventory management.

Thailand's vaccination program has faced challenges such as vaccine supply shortages, technical glitches, and public skepticism about the safety and efficacy of vaccines. To address these challenges, the government has increased vaccine procurement, launched a public information campaign to promote vaccine acceptance, and established a vaccine tracking system to monitor vaccine distribution.

An essential best practice observed in Thailand's VIS is the seamless integration of multiple data sources. The Mor Prom platform is linked to various databases, including national identification systems and electronic health records, ensuring accurate and up-to-date vaccination information. This integration has enabled health care providers to access comprehensive patient records and make informed decisions regarding vaccination eligibility and follow-up doses.

Thailand has also implemented proactive strategies to address vaccine hesitancy through VIS. The Mor Prom platform includes features that allow individuals to access reliable information about vaccines, including their safety and efficacy. The platform provides educational materials, frequently asked questions, and real-time updates on vaccine-related developments. By promoting transparent and accessible information, the app has helped build public trust and confidence in COVID-19 vaccines.

Thailand's VIS demonstrated a commitment to equitable vaccine distribution. The Mor Prom app incorporates an allocation algorithm that considers population density, vulnerability, and health care infrastructure to ensure the equitable, regional distribution of vaccines. This approach helps mitigate disparities and ensures equitable access to vaccination services across the country.

Furthermore, the success of Thailand's VIS can be attributed to strong leadership and collaboration between the government, health care providers, and technology partners, which has been instrumental in driving the implementation and adoption of digital health solutions. This collaboration has allowed continuous monitoring and evaluation of the system's performance, enabling timely adjustments and improvements to enhance user experience and address emerging challenges.

To further improve the country's VIS, ongoing efforts should focus on data interoperability and privacy protection. Interconnecting different health information systems and ensuring seamless data exchange can facilitate a more holistic view of individuals' health information and support comprehensive vaccination management. Additionally, robust data security measures and adherence to privacy regulations are crucial to maintaining public trust and confidence in the system.

Viet Nam

The country's electronic information systems include the National Immunization Information System (NIIS) and the COVID-19 Vaccination Portal. The NIIS is a digital platform developed by the Ministry of Health to manage and monitor the country's immunization programs. It is a centralized database that stores and manages individual vaccination records, vaccine inventory, and program data. It was used to manage vaccine distribution, track the number of vaccinated individuals, and generate vaccination reports. The NIIS supports functionalities such as registration, scheduling, and reporting to ensure efficient immunization management and monitoring. It allows for real-time monitoring of vaccine coverage and identifies immunization gaps, enabling targeted interventions and ensuring equitable access to vaccines.

Additionally, it enhances data accuracy, reduces paperwork, and facilitates data sharing among health care facilities. However, challenges such as interoperability, data privacy, and the digital divide still need to be addressed to maximize the system's potential and ensure its sustainability.

On the other hand, the COVID-19 Vaccination Portal was used to schedule vaccination appointments and provide vaccination information. An online platform similar to the one developed by the Ministry of Health, the portal allowed eligible individuals to register for vaccination, select vaccination sites, and receive appointment notifications. It also provided real-time updates on the availability of vaccines, vaccination progress, and adverse event reporting. The online platform improved accessibility, reduced manual paperwork, and enabled efficient resource allocation. It helped manage vaccine demand, prevented overcrowding at vaccination sites, and ensured a smooth vaccination experience for the population. However, the portal also encountered challenges such as internet access, digital literacy, and inclusivity for marginalized populations.

Another app developed to facilitate the country's COVID-19 response is PC-Covid Viet Nam, which consolidates into a single platform the various functionalities for vaccine certificates, travel permits, health declaration, and contact tracing. Its primary purpose has been to offer a COVID-19 card, a travel and social pass exclusively for individuals who are fully vaccinated against or have recovered from COVID-19. This card provides an official verification of a person's COVID-19 status, allowing them to engage in various activities with ease. One of the critical features of the PC-Covid Viet Nam app is the storage of a personal QR code that can be scanned to verify an individual's COVID-19 status. Additionally, the app records the user's movement to facilitate contact-tracing efforts, a crucial component in controlling the spread of the virus. Furthermore, the app enables users to conveniently complete health declaration forms, thereby streamlining the provision of essential health information for efficient monitoring and response by relevant authorities. The app also offers a map highlighting areas with high case numbers, providing users with crucial information to make informed decisions about their movements and potential exposure risks. Overall, the PC-Covid Viet Nam app serves as a reliable, centralized source of information related to COVID-19 vaccinations and the latest news regarding the pandemic.

However, when using apps like PC-Covid Viet Nam, it is crucial to consider factors such as data privacy, security, and user consent to ensure the protection of personal information. Transparent communication about data handling practices, adherence to data protection regulations, and user awareness campaigns are essential to building trust and encouraging widespread adoption of the application.

Relatedly, Viet Nam's vaccination program has faced challenges such as vaccine supply shortages, logistical constraints, and public skepticism about the safety and efficacy of vaccines. To address these challenges, the government has ramped up vaccine production and distribution, launched a public information campaign to promote vaccine acceptance, and established a vaccine passport system to facilitate international travel. The government has also collaborated with community leaders and influencers to promote vaccine uptake.

Viet Nam's experience integrating multiple health information systems into a single platform, as demonstrated by the PC-Covid app, highlights the importance of strong governance, collaboration among stakeholders, and clear communication strategies. These elements are essential for achieving seamless integration and maximizing the effectiveness of digital health solutions. The interoperability and integration of these systems, along with user-centric design, real-time data monitoring, and effective communication strategies, have yielded positive outcomes in Viet Nam's COVID-19 vaccination campaign.

Specifically, the PC-Covid Viet Nam app represents a significant advancement in the country's digital health ecosystem. With its multiple functionalities, it has served as a COVID-19 card, a travel pass, and a platform for health declaration, contact tracing, and information dissemination. Combining the strengths of existing systems such as the Viet Nam Health Declaration app, Bluetooth-powered contact-tracing app Bluezone, and the NCOVI app, this new app has led to a more cohesive and efficient approach to COVID-19 management.

Moreover, Viet Nam's VIS demonstrates the country's commitment to leveraging digital health technologies to enhance its COVID-19 response. Integrating various systems into the PC-Covid app has improved data exchange, streamlined processes, reduced systemic redundancy, and enhanced efficiency and user experience. Likewise, the NIIS, with its provision of real-time vaccination-related data, has led to timely and accurate decision-making by the authorities and service providers. Additionally, the accessible and user-friendly interfaces of these platforms highlight the importance of prioritizing users' needs and preferences to ensure inclusivity and maximize vaccine uptake.

By providing transparent and reliable information on COVID-19 vaccines, their safety, and effectiveness, these VISs have helped address vaccine hesitancy. Using such systems to disseminate evidence-based vaccine information is essential to building trust and confidence among the population and consequently increasing vaccine acceptance. In the long run, such systems also support the equitable distribution of vaccines, reducing disparities and promoting health equity.

Similarities and Differences of Vaccine Information Systems

Despite the differences in the implementation of VIS across the five DMCs, common factors are observable.

First is the use of digital platforms to facilitate vaccine registration, appointment scheduling, and monitoring. Digital platforms have the advantage of providing real-time data and enabling a rapid response to vaccine supply and demand. However, digital platforms also face challenges such as technical glitches, data privacy concerns, and unequal access to technology.

Second, the mobilization of unique QR codes to access vaccination records and monitor vaccine distribution and administration. This enables real-time monitoring of the vaccination program and can help identify areas where vaccine uptake is low.

Third, the use of vaccination certificates for travel and other purposes. Vaccination certificates serve as proof of vaccination and facilitate mobility. However, the use of vaccination certificates also raises issues such as data privacy, vaccine equity, and potential discrimination against unvaccinated individuals.

The fourth and final factor is the pursuit of communication campaigns to promote vaccine uptake and address vaccine hesitancy. In most countries, the government collaborates with health care providers and community leaders to promote vaccine uptake and provide accurate information. This is particularly important in areas with low health literacy and high rates of hesitancy.

Meanwhile, variations in the implementation of vaccine information systems across Southeast Asian countries reflect differences in the level of technological infrastructure, funding availability, and regulatory framework. Centralized and decentralized VIS have been implemented in different countries. For example, the Philippines and Indonesia have implemented centralized VIS, where data are collected and managed by a central agency; in contrast, Viet Nam and Cambodia have implemented decentralized systems, where data are collected and managed at the local level.

Another variation across the countries is the use of different types of VIS, such as web-based platforms, mobile applications, and digital health cards. The choice of VIS depends on factors such as digital infrastructure, resources, and the level of technology adoption in the population.

Another variation is the specific challenges encountered in implementing the VIS in each country. For example, Cambodia faced challenges related to limited digital infrastructure or low health literacy, while the Philippines, Indonesia, and Viet Nam faced challenges related to vaccine hesitancy or limited resources.

Despite these differences, the five DMCs have made significant efforts to integrate VIS into their COVID-19 response strategies. For instance, Thailand integrated its VIS into its national COVID-19 surveillance system to monitor vaccine distribution and adverse events following immunization. In the Philippines, vaccine information was used to identify priority groups for vaccination, such as health care workers and persons with comorbidities.

CHAPTER 4

Promoting Pharmacovigilance and Ensuring Vaccine Safety

KEY POINTS

- Although national regulatory authorities and pharmacovigilance systems were established decades before the pandemic, countries in the region calibrated these systems in response to COVID-19 to ensure the safety, quality, and efficacy of vaccines and other drugs.
- Evidence-based governance, public feedback mechanisms, efficient data management, and use of electronic reporting systems all contributed to high levels of regulatory maturity.
- The harmonization of regulatory systems across developing member countries will ensure that weak pharmacovigilance systems can draw best practices from the more established ones.
- Beyond ensuring the quality and safety of vaccines and pharmaceuticals, national regulatory authorities can also enhance efficiency and cost-effectiveness.

The COVID-19 pandemic precipitated a major paradigm shift in the global health agenda. International and national public health bodies quickly saw vaccination as the ultimate solution to the pandemic and calibrated their systems, priorities, and investments accordingly. The accelerating demands for COVID-19 vaccines were a major drive for changes in health systems and manufacturers worldwide. As of 1 October 2022, 12.7 billion doses had been given, and 68% of the world population had received at least one dose of COVID-19 vaccine.[60] Consequently, national regulatory authorities (NRA) and pharmacovigilance (PV) have become crucial for health systems to ensure the safety, quality, and efficacy of vaccines and other drugs being given to the public.

Although NRAs and PV systems were established decades before the pandemic, guidelines and standards for PV, adverse drug reactions (ADR), and adverse events following immunization (AEFI) surveillance have been diverse. The European Medicines Agency used Eudra-Vigilance; the US Food and Drug Administration (FDA)

[60] Our World in Data. 2022. *Coronavirus (COVID-19) Vaccination*, updated on 1 October 2022. https://ourworldindata.org/covid-vaccinations?country=OWID_WRL.

applied its Adverse Event Reporting System; and WHO used Vigi-Base. Similarly, many vaccines manufactured during the pandemic were in different phases of clinical evaluation. Although Europe and the US appeared well-positioned to implement vaccine safety programs at par with the pandemic's magnitude, scaling up regulatory authority, detecting adverse events, and minimizing risks became considerable challenges for other parts of the world.[61]

The Global Benchmarking Tool (GBT) for regulatory assessment, mandated by the World Health Assembly and released in 2016, was a game changer in assessing the maturity level of NRA systems worldwide in a standardized way. However, many countries overlooked their NRA capacity assessment to effectively and efficiently regulate vaccines and medicinal products before the pandemic.[62] The COVID-19 vaccination campaigns became the impetus for DMCs to assess the maturity levels of their respective PV systems. Correspondingly, these DMCs found the need to improve their maturity levels within a compressed interval, given the urgency of rolling out vaccination programs.

This chapter reviews how DMCs in Southeast Asia improved and promoted their PV systems during the pandemic. What were the enabling environments for PV systems, and what were the best practices? Answering these questions can contribute to strengthening such systems and meeting the accelerating demands for the safety of vaccines and other medical products.

This chapter uses the rapid assessment tools based on the WHO Global Benchmark Tool (2016) to review the NRA and PV systems of seven countries in Southeast Asia: Cambodia, Indonesia, the Lao PDR, the Philippines, Thailand, Timor-Leste, and Viet Nam. It uses available ADB documents, including country consultation missions and discussions with designated national focal persons of NRA and PV systems. It explores existing NRA and PV policies and regulations, reviews available standards, procedures and guidelines, and assesses various infrastructures and systems. Collating data from participatory consultative approaches with various stakeholders from PV and NRA systems of the listed countries, this chapter highlights the gaps and challenges in (i) policy, (ii) systems and procedures, and (iii) resources such as infrastructure, human resources, and technical and financial constraints.

---

61 WHO. 2022. *Pharmacovigilance of COVID-19 Vaccine*. https://www.who.int/groups/global-advisory-committee-on-vaccine-safety/topics/covid-19-vaccines/pharmacovigilance.

62 J. Guzman et al. 2020, The WHO Global Benchmarking Tool: A Game Changer for Strengthening National Regulatory Capacity. *BMJ Global Health. 5. e003181. 10.1136/bmjgh-2020-003181.*

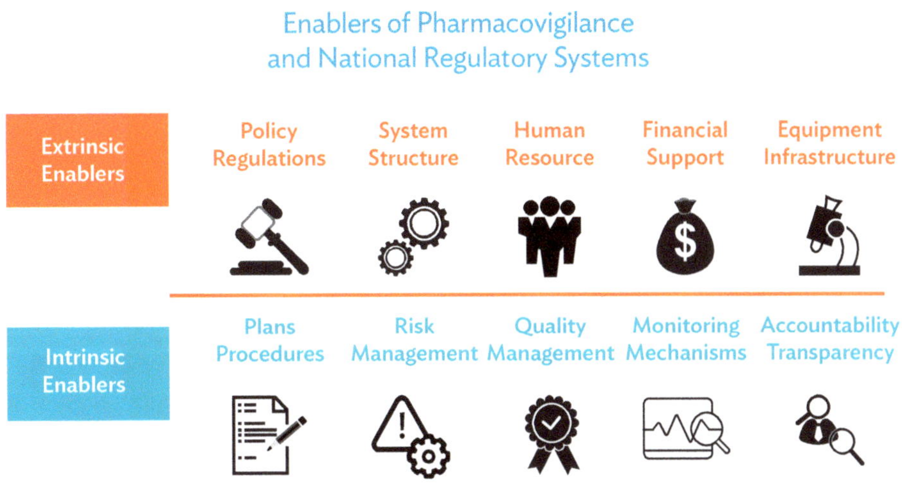

Source: Asian Development Bank. *Technical Assistance for Supporting Enhanced COVID-19 Vaccination and Post-COVID-19 Health Security Response in Southeast Asia.* https://www.adb.org/projects/55215-001/main (TA 6767-REG).

Framework: Enabling Improved Regulatory and Pharmacovigilance Systems

Regulatory authority and PV systems are generally managed by food and drug administrations. Scaling up the regulatory and PV system is a time-consuming and resource-intensive task. Therefore, the success of these systems depends on several enabling factors among responsible institutions, distinguishable into extrinsic and intrinsic factors. Intrinsic enablers are factors fulfilled by the system itself to improve its maturity. Setting up good plans and procedures, complying with risk management practices, installing quality management systems, and establishing accountability and transparency mechanisms are visible intrinsic factors for an enabling environment in NRA and PV systems. Extrinsic enablers are factors that enhance the system through external sources. As shown in the figure, enabling policy and regulation, establishing structures and organizations, employing adequate and skillful human resources, generating sustainable funding, and investing in infrastructure and technology are examples of key extrinsic enablers.

In analyzing the intrinsic enablers of DMCs, one can observe how many countries have established standards, plans, and procedures. However, the implementation of those standards has been limited, which has made scaling up good practices a major challenge. While countries with higher maturity levels (MLs) (levels 3 and 4) have focused on strengthening their monitoring and accountability systems, DMCs with less mature NRAs have faced many challenges in strengthening their systems. Partly, this is because scaling up intrinsic enablers is not only the responsibility of government, but also of various stakeholders—manufacturers, external assessors, prescribers, consumers, and academic institutions.

With regard to extrinsic enablers, almost all DMCs have promulgated policies, laws, and regulations related to regulatory authorities and drug control. However, many DMCs have faced persistent challenges in enforcing those regulations. Some have extended their PV and NRA structures beyond government institutions to involve academic institutions, manufacturers, nongovernment organizations, and consumer associations.[63] Another critical factor in strengthening NRA systems is human resource development. Many DMCs have a shortage of professionals skilled in PV, registration, risk management, post-marketing surveillance, authorization, and the administration of clinical trials in the regulatory system. Similarly, financial support and investment from domestic and overseas arenas have been lower for NRA and PV systems than other health systems services. Furthermore, regulatory systems need various structural and technological support, such as information technology (IT) platforms for data management, electronic systems for registration, licensing, and surveillance, and biotechnologies for laboratory and testing to ensure the quality, safety, and efficacy of medicinal products. Addressing these gaps and enhancing support for extrinsic enablers are critical to upgrading the maturity levels of NRA and PV systems.

Regional and Country Analyses Before and During the Pandemic

Rolling out vaccines requires well-established NRAs, robust PV platforms, good coordination of post-licensure surveillance, real-time information sharing, a robust data repository, and strong communication between countries.[64] Among the DMCs that are members of the Association of Southeast Asian Nations (ASEAN), a mutual recognition arrangement on good manufacturing practice inspection (MRA-GMP) was endorsed on 10 April 2009.[65] The MRA-GMP has been a priority roadmap for integrating ASEAN health sectors and regulatory authorities. During the pandemic, this MRA enabled mutual recognition and acceptance of GMP inspection reports and certification of COVID-19 vaccines and drugs among ASEAN DMCs, thereby saving time and resources for both regulators and manufacturers. The MRA not only facilitated better access to pharmaceuticals but also enhanced the standards and recognition of ASEAN GMP inspection services. Still, there remain considerable gaps for improvement with regard to achieving mutual agreements on vaccine and drug registration, risk management, PV, post-marketing surveillance, and distribution practices akin to those in European and North American countries.

Cambodia

Pre-pandemic. The Department of Drugs and Food (DDF) Essential Drugs Bureau managed the PV and NRA systems, which were chaired by the Secretary of State, Ministry of Health (MOH). The MOH issued Announcement No. 0973 in November 2011, requiring manufacturers and registration holders to submit ADR reports to DDF when they registered pharmaceuticals. DDF developed the national guidelines for ADR in August 2012, the guidelines for good storage practices in

63 V. Kalaiselvan et al. 2016. Pharmacovigilance Programme of India: Recent Developments and Future Perspectives. *Indian Journal of Pharmacology.* 48 (6). pp. 624–628. http://doi.org/10.4103/0253-7613.194855; L. Ratan and L. Mangala. 2015. An Update on the Pharmacovigilance Programme of India. *Frontiers in Pharmacology.* 6. 194. https://www.frontiersin.org/articles/10.3389/fphar.2015.00194.

64 D. Naniche et al. 2021. Beyond the Jab: A Need for Global Coordination of Pharmacovigilance for COVID-19 Vaccine Deployment. *eClinicalMedicine* 36. 100925. https://doi.org/10.1016/j.eclinm.2021.100925.

65 ASEAN. 2010. *ASEAN: Sectoral MRA for GMP Inspection of Manufactures of Medicinal Product.*

December 2015, and the guidelines for drug prescriptions in January 2017. In June 2015, DDF established the Cambodia Pharmacovigilance Centre, which distributed ADR reporting forms to health facilities for PV. However, ADRs were underreported because reporting was voluntary among health professionals. In August 2019, DDF developed a one-stop system for online registration of pharmaceuticals.

During the pandemic. DDF built an official website for public announcements on vaccine and drug safety and regularly published pharmaceutical statistics and regulatory decisions for the public. It used a QR code system through the Cambodia Pharmaceutical Online Registration System and had pages or channels on Facebook, Telegram, and YouTube. As of October 2022, eight COVID-19 vaccines were being marketed in the country.[66] However, despite the digitalization of the NRA, the PV advisory committee was nonfunctional during the pandemic, and no maturity level assessment has been conducted since. There was a severe shortage of human resources in national and provincial PV centers, the guidelines were outdated for at least a decade, and staff did not receive adequate PV training. Furthermore, the DDF had insufficient infrastructure to fulfill the various functions of a proper NRA.

Indonesia

Pre-pandemic. The advisory board and national program on ADR monitoring was established in 1980 through voluntary reporting by health workers. The National Agency of Drug and Food Control (Badan Pengawas Obat dan Makanan [BPOM]; since 2020 officially termed in English as the Indonesian Food and Drug Authority) became the country's chief NRA and joined the WHO drug monitoring program in 1990.In 2004, a PV unit was established under the Directorate of Distribution Control of Therapeutic and Household Healthcare Product, Ministry of Health. From 2008 to 2011, the country further strengthened legal frameworks, with the NRA releasing a series of degrees (1010/Menkes/Per/XI/2008 on drug registration, 1799/Menkes/Per/XXII/2010 on PV mandatory performance, and HK.03.1.23.12.11.10690 in 2011 for PV implementation, with technical guidelines for the pharmaceutical industry). The Good Manufacturing Practices (GMP) on drug manufacturing, published in 1989, was revised in 2001, 2005, and 2012.

The country's PV system consists of (i) voluntary reporting through hospitals, public health centers, general and private practices, and pharmacies; and (ii) mandatory reporting through the pharmaceutical industry and marketing authorization holders. The PV reporting flow begins with the patients or users through either a paper-based or an online system, proceeding to the use BPOM and then to the Uppsala Monitoring Center. Since 2010, BPOM has been conducting annual PV training and provides PV competency training for the pharmaceutical industry every 2 years. From 2012 to 2014, the NRA's functions were linked to the country's public health program, resulting in the decentralization of AEFI surveillance and electronic ADR reporting to provincial health departments (POM). Since then, POMs have functioned as PV centers and played vital roles in overseeing vaccine safety in the country. Despite the implementation of the Active Drug Safety Monitoring and Management in 2017, there is still considerable underreporting, insufficient information dissemination and awareness among the public, and a lack of formal feedback mechanisms in recognizing severe adverse events.

[66] COVID19 Vaccine Tracker. Cambodia, Updated 3 October 2022. https://covid19.trackvaccines.org/country/Cambodia/.

During the pandemic. In 2021, the country's NRA was assessed to be at ML-3. As of October 2022, 11 COVID-19 vaccines had been approved and 17 were undergoing clinical trials.[67] Twenty-eight POMs functioned as provincial PV centers during the pandemic. While POMs have developed references for implementing good PV practices and risk management plans, the challenges they continue to face include inadequate competency of and compliance with good PV practices among POM staff, as well as the lack of awareness of drug safety among manufacturers, prescribers, and the general public. Another challenge during the pandemic was the rampant illegal sale of prescription drugs in informal outlets (an estimated 5,000 unlicensed pharmacies and 90,000 informal outlets).[68] In 2020, the NADFC started the online application e-MESO for PV reporting; PV officers would verify reports in e-MESO and conduct causality assessments as necessary. By the following year, the system had received 8,691 ADR reports.[69] Additionally, the NADFC also made available the Drug Safety Rapid Alert System (DSRAS), which frequently provided updates on pharmaceutical safety information to the public.

Lao People's Democratic Republic

Pre-pandemic. The Food and Drug Department (FDD) piloted a PV project in 2012 with the support of WHO. In 2014, the FDD established a separate division to focus on PV system strengthening. In 2015, the country became a member of the WHO Programme for Drug Monitoring. In terms of legislation, the country had a robust legal system for medicine and drug control with Regulation on GMP 1999, National Medicine Policy 2003, and Drug and Medical Product Law 2004 (revised in 2012). Since 2015, training for PV and causality assessment has been provided with assistance from WHO. The annual ADR bulletin has also been published for the general public since 2012.

During the pandemic. FDD established the Vaccine Adverse Event Information Management, with its corresponding website. It also conducted a self-assessment of the NRA maturity level in 2021 and attained ML-2. As of October 2022, six COVID-19 vaccines had been approved in the country, while one was undergoing clinical trials.[70] Despite the website providing a venue for knowledge sharing and online registration of ADRs, FDD still needs to build capacity for online registration of pharmaceuticals. The country has limited capacity for vaccine distribution practices and post-marketing surveillance of pharmaceuticals.

Philippines

Pre-pandemic. The country's ADR reporting system was established in August 1994. In February 1995, the country was recognized as a member of the WHO international drug monitoring system. Meanwhile, Republic Act No. 9711, known as the Food and Drug Administration Act, authorized the country's FDA to prescribe guidelines and regulations pertaining to information on and marketing of pharmaceuticals. In 2014, the FDA also issued Circular 003/2014, which integrated the application form for the registration, certification, licensing, and compliance of good manufacturing practices to promote accountability and

---

67 COVID19 Vaccine Tracker. Indonesia, Updated 3 October 2022. https://covid19.trackvaccines.org/country/Indonesia/.

68 Y. Mahendradhata et al. 2017. The Republic of Indonesia Health System Review. *Health Systems in Transition*. 7 (1). https://apps.who.int/iris/handle/10665/254716.

69 Badan POM. 2022. *Buletin Berita MESO* 40(1). https://e-meso.pom.go.id/web/useruploads/images/1220701114135--9840D55E-CC2F-42E0-8C52-7DEC7CCE5538.pdf.

70 COVID19 Vaccine Tracker. Lao PDR, Updated 3 October 2022. https://covid19.trackvaccines.org/country/lao-peoples-democratic-republic/.

transparency. Separately, the PV section under FDA was designated the national PV center responsible for collating ADR reports from pharmaceutical companies, hospitals, health workers, patients, and public health programs. To strengthen the PV system, the FDA issued Circular 012/2018 for post-marketing surveillance requirements and Circular 003/2020 for guidelines for the pharmaceutical industry on mandatory PV and ADR reporting. In February 2015, the FDA participated in the first Asia Pacific Pharmacovigilance Training Course in collaboration with the Uppsala Monitoring Center.

During the pandemic. The FDA issued Circular 029/2020 for the conduct of COVID-19 clinical trials, Circular 008/2021 for the registration of pharmaceuticals under emergency use, Circular 025/2021 for the authorization to use said pharmaceuticals in light of the state of public health emergency, Circular 004/2022 for the establishment of registration pathways for pharmaceuticals, and Circular 005/2022 for the requirement to label pharmaceuticals under maximum retail prices. The FDA also conducted a self-assessment of the NRA using the WHO GBT in 2020 and attained ML-1-2. As of July 2022, the FDA had authorized nine COVID-19 vaccines for emergency use. In collaboration with the Department of Health, the FDA also established a reporting system of suspected AEFI of COVID-19 vaccines based on the national VigiFlow database. From 1 March 2021 to 10 July 2022, 104,211 suspected ADR reports were received, evaluated, and analyzed by that system.[71] Despite the established integrated IT platform for vaccine and drug registration and quality assurance, the FDA is challenged by the inadequate interoperability of its electronic system. There has also been under-reporting of ADRs, requiring improvements to digitalizing this PV system.

Thailand

Pre-pandemic. The country established its NRA, national PV center, and PV system in 1983 before joining the WHO drug monitoring and reporting system the following year. In 2010, the country shifted its PV focus from hospital-based to community-based ADR monitoring for all drug-related problems. The Thai FDA adopted good PV and risk management practices from the EMA, US FDA, and Pharmaceutical and Medical Devices Agency-Japan. It also established an online platform system for the registration and licensing of pharmaceuticals. The Thai Vigibase online reporting and surveillance system was established to collect ADR reports from various sources, including hospitals, pharmacies, and clinics.

During the pandemic. In collaboration with WHO, NRA maturity was assessed based on the WHO GBT criteria in 2021. The country achieved ML-3 for vaccines. As of October 2022, seven COVID-19 vaccines had been approved by NRA Thailand and 12 were undergoing clinical trials.[72] Despite its ML-3 assessment, the Thai FDA still faced difficulties harmonizing ADR reports from various information sources, with identifiable gaps and challenges in data flow from provincial to national reporting units. As such, the Thai FDA has sought to strengthen good PV and risk management practices beyond government agencies to include manufacturers, the private sector, and the academe, hopefully to increase its maturity level to ML-4. Part of its efforts included a nationwide awareness campaign on vaccine safety and

[71] Government of the Philippines, Food and Drug Administration. 2022. *Reports of Suspected Adverse Reaction to COVID-19 Vaccines (01 March 2021 to 10 July 2022).* https://www.fda.gov.ph/wp-content/uploads/2022/03/Reports-of-suspected-adverse-reaction-to-COVID-19-vaccines-as-of-13-March-2022.pdf.

[72] COVID19 Vaccine Tracker. Thailand, Updated 3 October 2022. https://covid19.trackvaccines.org/country/thailand/.

vaccine distribution that was done alongside the vaccinations. It can be said that the country (and its FDA in particular) has been actively promoting good vaccine distribution practices for a post-COVID-19 world.

Timor-Leste

Pre-pandemic. There was no official NRA in the country. Some NRA functions were fulfilled by the National Directorate of Pharmacy and Medicines, which oversaw licensing, PV, and market authorization. The Department of Pharmacy was responsible for the management and quantification of vaccines and drugs at health facilities. At the same time, the Service Autonomo de Medicamentos e Equipamentos de Saude was responsible for the procurement and supply of all pharmaceuticals in public health facilities. Post-licensing inspections, including for commercial pharmacies, were conducted by the Cabinet of Inspection, an independent body answerable to the Vice Minister for Health. In 2010, the National Drug Act and the National Drug and Medicine Policy were promulgated. The National Standard Treatment Guidelines were updated in 2010, while the National Essential Medicine List was revised in 2015.

During the pandemic. Major challenges in the pharmaceutical sector concerned drug supply, selection, regulation, and information dissemination, with poor manual inventory control systems at municipal hospitals. With no technical committee for drug registration and PV, the country could not establish a formal ADR monitoring and reporting system. However, with technical assistance from UNICEF and WHO, the national immunization program established an AEFI reporting system for COVID-19 vaccines. In 2021, the National Directorate of Pharmacy and Medicines conducted a consultative workshop with private pharmacies, clinics, and drug importers to develop the country's first PV guidelines. The draft guidelines were developed with technical assistance from WHO and presented to the Council of Directors for approval.

Viet Nam

Pre-pandemic. The country's NRA and PV systems were built through legislation comprising the Law on Pharmacy 105/2016/QH13; Decree 54/2017/ND-CP for implementation of guidelines; Decree 104/2016/ND-CP for safety of vaccination; Circular 29/2018/TT-BYT on clinical trials; and Circular 51/2017/TT-BYT for guidelines on prevention, diagnosis, and management of anaphylaxis and warnings about ADRs. Drug Administration Viet Nam (DAV), helmed by the Vice Minister for Health, oversees the country's NRA and PV systems. DAV established two ADR centers at the University of Pharmacy, Ha Noi, and Cho Ray Hospital in Ho Chi Minh City. It also has a website with a registration system and regular announcements of vaccine and drug evaluation reports. As of 31 December 2019, 68 vaccines had market authorization in the country.

During the pandemic. The NRA underwent two maturity level assessments: first in 2015 and then in 2020, when it attained ML-3. DAV continues to face many challenges regarding the amendment of regulations, human resources for NRAs, drug pricing, data management and digitalization, and evaluation of vaccine registration dossiers. Throughout the pandemic, DAV encountered gaps in communication between their website and mobile operators for online registration and ADR reporting. Nonetheless, with its strict reporting and surveillance system, the country accounted for 22,265 cases of normal and 46 cases of severe reactions after vaccine injections in 2020. As of October 2022, eight COVID-19 vaccines had been approved, and nine were undergoing clinical trials in the country.[73]

In 2021, the country's NRA was assessed at ML-3. As of October 2022, 11 COVID-19 vaccines had been approved, and 17 were undergoing clinical trials.[74] Twenty-eight POMs functioned as provincial PV centers during the pandemic. While POMs have developed references for implementing good PV practices and risk management plans, the challenges they continue to face include inadequate competency of and compliance with good PV practices among POM staff, as well as the lack of awareness of drug safety among manufacturers, prescribers, and the general public. Another challenge during the pandemic was the rampant illegal sale of prescription drugs in informal outlets (an estimated 5,000 unlicensed pharmacies and 90,000 informal outlets) (footnote 68). In 2020, the NADFC started the online application e-MESO for PV reporting; PV officers would verify reports in e-MESO and conduct causality assessments as necessary. By the following year, the system had received 8,691 ADR reports (footnote 69). The NADFC also made available the Drug Safety Rapid Alert System, which frequently provided updates on pharmaceutical safety information to the public.

Good Practices for National Regulatory Authorities and Pharmacovigilance During the Pandemic

Amid the paradigm shift in the global health agenda, many countries took the opportunity to improve their NRA and PV systems during the pandemic. Table 3 is an overview of the status of regulatory authorities in seven DMCs.

Governance

Evidence-based governance is one of the good practices for scaling NRAs. The Global Vaccine Safety Blueprint 2021–2023 was developed collaboratively by WHO and its PV partners during the pandemic, providing more inclusive strategies that DMCs could easily adopt to improve their vaccine safety systems. Furthermore, the blueprint enables regulatory frameworks to surveil AEFI and communicate vaccine safety among the general public more efficiently.[75] Another good governance practice was the regulatory convergence and reliance among ASEAN countries on the APEC harmonization strategic framework, enabling DMCs to improve regulatory agility by applying nontraditional approaches to regulatory decision-making without compromising the safety, quality, and efficacy of pharmaceuticals.[76]

---

73 COVID19 Vaccine Tracker. Viet Nam, Updated 3 October 2022. https://covid19.trackvaccines.org/country/viet-nam/.

74 COVID19 Vaccine Tracker. Indonesia, Updated 3 October 2022. https://covid19.trackvaccines.org/country/Indonesia/.

75 WHO. 2022. *Global Vaccine Safety Blueprint 2.0 2021-2023.* https://apps.who.int/iris/rest/bitstreams/1392676/retrieve.

76 APEC. 2021. Strategic Framework Regulatory Harmonization Steering Committee Vision 2030 and Strategic Framework Regulatory Convergence for Medical Products by 2030. https://www.apec.org/docs/default-source/satellite/RHSC/General-RHSC-Documents/APEC-RHSCVision-2030-and-Strategic-Framework-2021-Jan.pdf.

Table 3: Status of National Regulatory Authorities Among Seven Developing Member Countries in Southeast Asia

Country	National Regulatory Authority	ML	Status of Assessment	Gaps and Challenges
Thailand	Thailand Food and Drug Administration	3	GBT-2021 ADB-2022	Risk management, distribution, and ADR reporting, monitoring
Viet Nam	Drug Administration Viet Nam (DAV)	3	GBT-2021 ADB-2022	Risk management, registration, drug pricing, and digitalization
Indonesia	Indonesian Food and Drug Authority (BPOM)	3	GBT-2021	
Lao PDR	Food and Drug Department (FDD)	2	GBT-2021 ADB-2022	Registration, IEC, post-market surveillance, and risk management
Philippines	Philippine Food and Drug Administration	1	GBT-2021	
Cambodia	Department of Drugs and Food (DDF)	1	ADB-2022	PV, supply chain management, digitalization
Timor-Leste	National Directorate of Pharmacy and Medicines	1	ADB-2022	PV, procurement and distribution, risk mitigation

ADB = Asian Development Bank; ADR = adverse drug reaction; BPOM = Badan Pengawas Obat dan Makanan; GBT = global benchmarking tool; IEC = information education, and communication; Lao PDR = Lao People's Democratic Republic; ML = maturity level; NRA = national regulatory authority; PV = pharmacovigilance; WHO = World Health Organization.
Sources: WHO Global Benchmarking Tool (2016) (GBT-2021); SECURE Project Tools to identify NRA gaps (ADB-2022).

Regulatory Framework

Regulatory authorities need to establish a coherent, flexible, and responsive regulatory framework that considers the limitation of resources, public expectations, and the occurrence of large-scale health emergencies. The Health Sciences Authority of Singapore achieved ML-4 by addressing public trust and responsiveness to its regulatory system during the pandemic.[77] HAS established public feedback mechanisms and released safety reports on COVID-19 vaccines and other drugs on a monthly basis. Furthermore, complying with international audit standards, the Singapore FDA established flexible internal monitoring mechanisms to address the changes caused by public health emergencies. Thailand and Viet Nam also reviewed their regulatory frameworks during the pandemic and improved NRA capacity to reach ML-3.

Biosafety Technologies

Achieving local manufacturing capacity for COVID-19 vaccines has become a goal for many countries, regardless of existing technical and regulatory capacities for vaccine manufacturing. Since the minimum efficacy of COVID-19 vaccines is more than 50%, it can be challenging for biopharmaceutical industries to hasten vaccine development timelines without compromising biosafety. One good practice is applying cutting-edge technology, such as next-generation sequencing technology for biosafety, which reduces the lead time for vaccine development and increases the confidence level of test results for biosafety testing compared

[77] M. Xu et al. 2022. Regulatory Reliance for Convergence and Harmonisation in the Medical Device Space in Asia-Pacific. *BMJ Global Health*. 7. e009798. https://gh.bmj.com/content/7/8/e009798.

with traditional testing techniques.[78] During the pandemic, manufacturers and regulatory agencies that used this technology shortened their lead times for vaccine development and safety monitoring. The National Vaccine Institute and Chulalongkorn University Thailand used such techniques to develop mRNA vaccines. Collaborating with the ASEAN Secretariat, the National Vaccine Institute hosted the Vaccine Network Consultation Meeting in September 2022 to disseminate its good practices on vaccine manufacturing, empowering research and policy development across the region.

Electronic Reporting

Increasing the availability of electronic records makes ADR reporting more efficient and can enable the real-time detection of vaccine and drug safety signals online. The EU-ADR Project (2008–2013) generated an extraordinary resource base for drug safety monitoring in Europe (30 million people from various institutions were involved).[79] That project demonstrated a previously unseen potential for ADR monitoring among the general population. During the pandemic, many DMCs upgraded their ADR/AEFI reporting systems by merging country data with global data through the WHO Vigiflow System. Indonesia and Thailand upgraded their reporting systems from paper-based to electronic, saving time and reducing the workload of health workers tasked to report AEFI of COVID-19 vaccines. Other countries such as Cambodia, the Lao PDR, and Viet Nam were in transitional stages (i.e., using paper-based systems at the district level but digitizing the data at the provincial level and beyond). Many countries were able to disseminate AEFI information on COVID-19 vaccination to the general public more efficiently through outreach immunization and reporting services.

Data Management

Since PV primarily involves the collection, processing, and evaluation of case reports to detect and confirm ADRs, data management has played a significant role throughout the pandemic. Using artificial intelligence to manage big data has been a good practice for manufacturers and health facilities during the paradigm shift.[80] Singapore and the Republic of Korea installed big-data artificial intelligence systems for data storage, analysis, and visualization for PV during the pandemic. These countries also linked their respective systems to social media platforms to keep the public informed of data and decisions related to PV and pharmaceutical regulation. Meanwhile, Thailand and Viet Nam are scaling up NRA data management and data processing by synchronizing their digital information systems and investing in artificial intelligence technology for big-data management. Such investments can reduce the burden on health professionals and make systems more alert,

---

78 C. Côté and A. Brussel. 2021. COVID-19: Leading the Paradigm Shift in Biosafety Testing. *Pharmaceutical Outsourcing*, 6 September. https://www.pharmoutsourcing.com/Featured-Articles/579098-COVID-19-Leading-the-Paradigm-Shift-in-Biosafety-Testing/.

79 V. K. Patadia et al. 2015. Using Real-World Healthcare Data for Pharmacovigilance Signal Detection—The Experience of the EU-ADR Project. *Expert Review of Clinical Pharmacology.* 8 (1). pp. 95–102. https://www.tandfonline.com/doi/abs/10.1586/17512433.2015.992878?journalCode=ierj20.

80 A. Togra and S. Pawar. 2022. Role of Automation, Natural Language Processing, Artificial Intelligence, and Machine Learning in Hospital Settings to Identify and Prevent Adverse Drug Reactions. *Journal of Pharmacovigilance and Drug Research.* 3 (3). https://www.jpadr.com/index.php/jpadr/article/view/102.

thereby reducing preventable ADRs.[81] Although most DMCs are unprepared to advance toward artificial intelligence, the pandemic has shown the importance of investing in strengthening data management systems.

Conclusion

The diversity of maturity levels in the Southeast Asian region necessitates a more strategic approach to scaling up NRAs to reach acceptable standards. Like the ASEAN mutual recognition of good manufacturing practices, regional standards for good PV practices, risk management practices, post-marketing surveillance, and good vaccine distribution practices are required for all concerned DMCs. Currently, there are no tangible regional mechanisms or platforms for NRAs, nor is there a regional network for knowledge sharing on PV. A regional working group for NRA should be established with designated national focal points and specific functions. Such a network will be required for collaboration among the ASEAN's vaccine safety networks. Moreover, the engagement of regional policy actors is urgently required to map out strategic directions and structure the investment frameworks for scaling up the NRAs and PV systems in the region.

Harmonizing regulatory systems across DMCs will ensure that weak PV systems can draw best practices from the more established ones. Countries like Indonesia, Thailand, and Viet Nam are now in a transitional stage (ML-3) and can look toward investing further in cutting-edge technologies and public accountability mechanisms. Other DMCs are still in fundamental stages requiring various forms of support (e.g., technical assistance, longer-term infrastructure investments). Thus, a stepwise approach to strengthening national PV infrastructure based on available resources is required. Additionally, in building capacity for NRA and PV, national vaccine strategies and drug policies must be considered.

Manufacturers and market authorization holders in NRA systems have been engaged through regulations compatible with international standards.[82] Singapore reached ML-4 by complying with international FDA audit standards. Other countries, however, established their NRA systems decades ago with now obsolete guidelines. Given that the pandemic has transformed the health agenda, DMCs must adapt their organizational structures and revise those guidelines. The pandemic heavily influenced guidelines and procedures such as good PV, risk management, distribution practices and marketing surveillance, requiring mandatory revision for a post-COVID-19 world. These revisions should aim to create a culture where PV is prioritized, training programs on regulatory control and PV are embedded in pre-service and in-service training curricula, and training staff have easy access to up-to-date information.

---

[81] S. Lee et al. 2022. Hybrid Method Incorporating a Rule-Based Approach and Deep Learning for Prescription Error Prediction. *Drug Safety.* 45. pp. 27–35. https://link.springer.com/article/10.1007/s40264-021-01123-6.

[82] R. Kiguba et al. 2023. Pharmacovigilance in Low- and Middle-Income Countries: A Review with Particular Focus on Africa. *British Journal of Clinical Pharmacology.* 89 (2). pp. 491–509. https://bpspubs.onlinelibrary.wiley.com/doi/full/10.1111/bcp.15193.

PV systems in many developed countries are well-established not only at the national level but also at subnational and community levels. In contrast, the DMCs tackled in this chapter have focused mainly on strengthening only the national capacity of NRAs. There are considerable knowledge and resource gaps in subnational PV units and scaling them up is essential to ensuring the quality and safety of pharmaceuticals.

Since regulation involves various government departments, improving and sustaining cross-sectoral and intergovernmental communications are required. Clear policy implications in terms of promulgating and amending legislation can further promote accountability among concerned bodies. Countries should thus consider mandatory planning and budgeting to sustain NRA coordination mechanisms, including in times of health crises.

Public trust is crucial in unlocking the obstacles to improving regulatory systems in the era of social media and COVID-19. Therefore, quick, transparent, and responsive feedback mechanisms for PV-related incidents should now be accessible to health care workers, policymakers, and consumers. Targeted awareness campaigns and risk communications in DMCs can also promote awareness of PV and improve public trust in the health system.

Lastly, local vaccine development and manufacturing has inarguably become a dream for many countries. To counter potential overspending, regulatory authorities will be instrumental in safeguarding processes and providing evidence-based information not only to ensure the quality and safety of pharmaceuticals but also to share scarce resources more efficiently and reduce unnecessary waste among various health systems. As countries recover from the pandemic, NRAs will no doubt acquire an ever-larger role in bridging policymakers, manufacturers, and the general public in future vaccine manufacturing and development.

CHAPTER 5

Mobilizing Public–Private Partnerships

KEY POINTS

- Governments turned to public–private partnerships (PPPs) as a way to meet the immense challenges posed by the pandemic
- Common enablers of private sector engagement include a commitment to universal health care, high levels of donation-based PPPs, and robust regulatory frameworks.
- Moving forward, it is necessary to create enabling policy environments that balance the interests of both public and private partners, while maintaining inclusive development and public health goals as key shared priorities.

At the height of the COVID-19 pandemic, public health care systems across Asia were strained to their limits, undermined by preexisting infrastructure challenges to health service delivery. However, governments were also forced to react quickly and decisively by establishing health security interventions (HSIs) to curb the coronavirus' spread. Within this context, the private sector became pivotal to building that capacity, offering innovation, dynamism, and scaling benefits.

Public–private partnerships (PPPs) in the health sector are nothing new, but they have often been prioritized less than large-scale energy, infrastructure, or construction projects. In recent years, this perspective has shifted as governments looked for alternative strategies to finance health care infrastructure and services amid the rising costs of health provision. In developing countries, governments have come to view PPPs as desirable in building essential public health infrastructure and services and, in some cases, have included PPPs in their national strategy for health care. This need has become only more apparent during the pandemic.

The PPP experience during the pandemic varied across countries. Yet, among the six Southeast Asian countries, a common pattern emerged: more PPPs materialized in countries with stronger and more well-developed enabling environments. Drawing from a single-country analysis of each developing member country (DMC), this chapter presents some of the best practices in the region in terms of realizing PPPs, followed by recommendations that may be adopted by other countries.

This chapter defines PPPs broadly as encapsulating a range of possible relationships and engagements among the public (e.g., government entities such as ministries, departments, agencies, municipalities, and state-owned enterprises) and private (e.g., businesses, investors, multilateral bodies, development banks, donor countries, nongovernment organizations, and nonprofit organizations) entities. The service provided by a PPP is typically that of a state's responsibility but provided by the private partner under the terms of the partnership. This includes more traditional forms of PPPs such as build–operate–transfer, joint ventures, civil works and contracts, and partnerships established in the spirit of PPPs such as procurement, donations, and capacity building.

In particular, this chapter examines PPPs in three categories and eight subcategories of HSIs during the pandemic for six DMCs: Cambodia, Indonesia, the Lao PDR, the Philippines, Thailand, and Timor-Leste. The three categories are COVID-19 vaccinations, public health surveillance, and COVID-19 testing. These categories were selected because they have been prominent interventions during the pandemic and probable areas for PPPs to materialize.

The first category, COVID-19 vaccinations, encompasses (i) research and development; (ii) manufacturing; (iii) delivery of vaccinations; (iv) vaccination program management, including the use of databases, statistics, logistics, and coordination; and (v) vaccine risk communications and public education. The second category, public health surveillance, includes (i) movement tracking and contact tracing, including the use of smartphone applications to track movement and manage data; and (ii) epidemiological or disease modeling, wherein data is used through either artificial intelligence and machine learning systems to predict or manage outbreaks and disease clusters. Lastly, the third category, COVID-19 testing, includes laboratory support for testing provided by private laboratories, private hospitals, or private clinics, using both polymerase chain reaction (PCR) and antigen rapid test kits.

This chapter used a mixed-methods methodology to identify and assess PPPs and HSIs before and during the pandemic in the six DMCs. This entailed a systematic review of publicly available online and offline documents, including government press statements, official documents, academic journals, and news sources. Key informant interviews with public health experts based in or working on the six DMCs complemented the findings from this review. The semi structured interview format ensured consistent surveying while also maintaining flexibility to gather unanticipated information and allow for follow-up questions.

This data informed a larger report, which included single-country analyses. This chapter presents the more synthetic and applied aspects of that report, hopefully offering practical guidance as countries continue to look to PPPs as significant parts of their health care systems (Table 4).

Public–Private Partnerships in the Region: A Comparative Overview

Based on PPP Knowledge Lab data (Table 4), a large disparity exists in the number of PPP infrastructure projects between the first group of countries (Thailand, Indonesia, and the Philippines) and the second (the Lao PDR, Cambodia, and Timor-Leste). Thailand, Indonesia, and the Philippines each have more than 140 infrastructure PPPs that have reached financial closure since 1990, far more than the combined number for the Lao PDR, Cambodia, and Timor-Leste. Notably, Timor-Leste, which achieved independence in 2002, has recorded just three PPP infrastructure projects reaching financial closure.

Table 4: Snapshot of Public–Private Partnership Data and Other Macroeconomic and Health Indicators per Developing Member Country

Item	Thailand	Indonesia	Philippines	Lao PDR	Cambodia	Timor-Leste
COVID-19 HSI PPP and public–private collaboration (including procurement)						
Total COVID-19 HSI PPP initiatives	38	26	21	3	20	22
Of which: traditional procurement	7	4	6	NF	1	20
COVID-19 HSI PPPs, excluding procurement	31	22	15	3	19	2
Standalone private initiatives	3	1	1	NF	8	NF
PPP investment in infrastructure (PPP Knowledge Lab)						
Total Investment in PPP (USD million)	44,076	74,161	59,848	23,658	4,419	490
Total PPP projects	185	145	173	34	34	3
Macroeconomic indicators						
GDP (current USD millions)	501.6	1,058.4	361.5	19.1	25.8	1.9
GDP per capita	7,186.9	3,869.6	3,298.8	2,629.7	1,543.7	1,442.7
Tax revenue (% of GDP)	14.6	9.8	14.5	NF	19.7	22.6
World Bank income classification (2022)	Upper middle	Lower middle	Lower middle	Lower middle	Lower middle	Lower middle
Health care systems						
Current health expenditure (% of GDP)	3.8	2.9	4.1	2.6	7.0	7.2
Domestic private health expenditure (% of current health expenditure)	28.2	50.5	59.0	41.9	69.2	13.1
Universal Healthcare Service Coverage Index (2019)	83	59	55	50	61	53
Governance						
Corruption Perception Index	35	38	33	30	23	41
BTI Governance Index	4.0	5.2	4.3	4.2	3.1	5.8

BTI = Bertelsmann Stiftung Transformation, COVID-19 = coronavirus disease, GDP = gross domestic product, HSI = health security intervention, Lao PDR = Lao People's Democratic Republic, NF = not found, PPP = public–private partnership.

Notes: PPP investment data has been since 1990. All data points are the most recent available period.

Sources: World Bank. PPP Knowledge Lab; BTI Project Organization. The Transformation Index; ADB. 2022. *Report on Public–Private Partnerships in COVID-19 Vaccination Programs and Health Security Interventions in Six Developing Member Countries.*

Common Enablers of Private Sector Engagement in the Six Developing Member Countries

Common enabling factors among the six DMCs stood out as key contributors to private sector engagement. Notwithstanding country-specific circumstances and individual political economy considerations, this section highlights those enabling factors.

Recognition of the Importance of Public–Private Partnerships

All six DMCs share a common PPP philosophy that acknowledges the importance of PPPs in accelerating public infrastructure, with all countries exhibiting similar national goals of attracting more PPPs for development, albeit to varying levels of strategic and political commitment. Prior to the pandemic, PPPs had proven beneficial to upscaling health systems capacity and financing in these countries. This recognition of the centrality of PPPs to development comprises a core attribute of a robust enabling environment. Thus, during the pandemic, the countries that were more strongly committed to their own PPP philosophies boasted more PPPs and were able to improve, enhance, and expand their pandemic responses more effectively and efficiently.

However, there were differences among the enabling environments of the six DMCs. Not all countries had standalone governing or coordinating bodies dedicated to PPPs. Countries like Cambodia, the Lao PDR, Thailand, and Timor-Leste had specific units usually under the purview of their respective Ministries of Finance, while Indonesia and the Philippines created authoritative bodies focused solely on PPP facilitation. Thus, while national PPP philosophies could be responsive to and in favor of PPPs in general, the implementation differed and resulted in varying maturity levels of the enabling environment.

Commitment to Universal Health Coverage

Universal health coverage remains a key development goal of the six DMCs, with some countries having already established a universal health program and others still in the development stage. In terms of implementation, the Universal Healthcare Service Coverage Index scores across all countries are almost the same, with the exception of Thailand's relatively high score (Table 4). This score can be viewed as setting the stage for PPPs in HSIs and health service delivery in the six DMCs.

High Levels of Donation-Based Public–Private Partnerships

In many DMCs, PPPs during the pandemic were based mainly on donations from the private sector to build up HSI capacity in a bid to reopen the economy sooner, which was likely a response to the unique nature of the pandemic. The gains from these private sector engagements were usually indirect, such as prestige, influence, or publicity. However, successful partnerships were usually the result of arrangements that accorded mutual benefits for all parties involved.[83] Since PPPs that provided one-sided benefits would unlikely be successful in the long run, their sustainability remains in question (footnote 81).

[83] M. Mitchell. 2008. An Overview of PPPs in Health. *International Health Systems Program Publication, Harvard School of Public Health.*

However, across most of the DMCs, the pandemic undoubtedly catalyzed the pivot of national interest toward attracting more PPPs in health care service delivery instead of just primarily in transport or energy infrastructure, making it likely that more PPPs in HSIs or general health service delivery will materialize in the near future.

Robustness of Regulatory Frameworks

Regulatory PPP frameworks have been present in all DMCs, although some (e.g., Indonesia, the Philippines, Thailand) are more well-established than others, with the frameworks of Cambodia and the Lao PDR being the most recently developed. The levels of success have also been variable; Cambodia, the Lao PDR, and Timor-Leste have seen relatively limited success in attracting PPPs for the development of public infrastructure. Arguably, these three countries had less robust frameworks in place and less experience with PPPs compared to their regional counterparts, likely contributing to their difficulty in leveraging the private sector's potential for HSIs during the pandemic.

During the pandemic, countries with robust legal frameworks were better positioned to tap into the benefits of PPPs to manage the pandemic and leverage related opportunities. One explanation may be that the comprehensiveness of the frameworks allowed the private sector to identify a role for themselves in helping achieve public health objectives. For example, in Thailand, where the legal framework was first introduced in 1992, there were 38 PPPs during the pandemic, including those for the research and development, clinical trials, and manufacture of vaccines. Similarly, Indonesia had 26 PPPs, including a private sector vaccination drive, while the Philippines had 21, including a multi-stakeholder vaccine delivery program.

In contrast, countries with relatively newer or less-developed PPP legal frameworks had not only fewer PPPs but also PPPs that were often limited to capacity building, training, and procurement. For example, Timor-Leste had no specific PPP law until 2021, and its PPPs during the pandemic comprised predominantly of procurement contracts and capacity building. The same can be said of Cambodia, which also had no specific PPP law until 2021 and where ad hoc donations from business tycoons composed nearly half of PPPs during the pandemic. Meanwhile, aside from the PPPs developing a contact-tracing application and one vaccine trial, the other PPPs in the Lao PDR were limited to receiving a container lab to boost national testing capacity.

Country Best Practices

Cambodia

The country's PPP experience hints at the importance of a consultative process in formulating and establishing new laws. For instance, the drafting process of the country's 2021 PPP law included multiple consultative workshops with many stakeholders, including national ministries responsible for PPPs, development partners, law firms, banks, investors, insurance companies, construction companies, chambers of commerce, embassy representatives and private sector partners implementing existing PPP or concession contracts.[84]

---

[84] UNESCAP. 2020. *Cambodia: Current PPP Development.* https://www.unescap.org/sites/default/d8files/event-documents/Cambodia_PPP%20Management%20Framework%20Final%20v1.pdf.

Furthermore, the 2021 PPP law was prepared on the basis of the Policy Paper on PPPs for Public Investment Project Management 2016–2020, which was produced through a similar consultative process involving the ADB.[85]

Considering Cambodia's level of development, the country's reliance on development partners was expected. However, Cambodia's experience remains unique. During the pandemic, the existing PPP between the Government of Cambodia and the Institut Pasteur du Cambodge (IPC) led to the IPC becoming one of the main national laboratories for testing COVID-19 samples.[86] In recognition of the quality and importance of the work conducted by the IPC, WHO designated it as an International Reference Laboratory for COVID-19 to provide referral services, capacity building, data management and analysis, and viral culture and sequencing functions.[87]

Indonesia

Over the last 2 decades, Indonesia has demonstrated a commitment to private sector engagement and an incremental improvement of its PPP regulatory frameworks. Through these efforts, it was able to compensate for early missteps in its pandemic response by tapping the private sector to improve vaccine delivery, support tracking and tracing efforts, and increase capacity during the worst COVID-19 surges.

Efforts to improve the enabling and regulatory environment for PPPs proved critical. In the mid-2000s, Indonesia started enacting reforms to bolster private sector involvement not only in infrastructure development but also in other services like health care provision. The country enacted its first PPP regulation governing cooperation between the government and private entities in 2005 (Presidential Regulation No. 67/2005). Since then, this regulation has been amended thrice (2010, 2011, 2013) and, most recently, revised by Presidential Regulation 38/2015 (on Cooperation between Government and Business Entity in Infrastructure Provisioning).[88] Moreover, to overcome the structural challenges of PPP governance, Indonesia created the Infrastructure Guarantee Fund in 2009, lowering the risk and cost of financing. In 2017, it also established the PPP Joint Office to improve interagency coordination.

Described by the Organisation for Economic Co-operation and Development as a work in progress,[89] the country's focus on improving its PPP framework, as well as its commitment to leveraging private sector involvement for development has translated to a long working relationship between private firms and the public sector and ministries. This relationship and sustained engagement enabled the private sector to play a significant role in bolstering public

---

85 OECD. 2018. *OECD Investment Policy Reviews: Cambodia 2018. Paris.* https://www.oecd-ilibrary.org/finance-and-investment/oecd-investment-policy-reviews-cambodia_9789264309074-en.

86 B. Nit et al. 2021. Understanding the Slow COVID-19 Trajectory of Cambodia. *Public Health in Practice.* 2. https://www.sciencedirect.com/science/article/pii/S2666535220300720#bib12.

87 Institut Pasteur du Cambodge. 2020. Institut Pasteur du Cambodge Receives Designation as WHO International Reference Laboratory for COVID-19. https://www.pasteur-kh.org/2020/04/10/institut-pasteur-du-cambodge-receives-designation-as-who-international-reference-laboratory-for-covid-19/#:~:text=TEACHING-,Institut%20Pasteur%20du%20Cambodge%20receives%20designation%20as,Reference%20Laboratory%20for%20COVID%2D19&text=The%20World%20Health%20Organization%20(WHO,Reference%20Laboratory%20for%20COVID%2D19. Accessed 14 June 2022.

88 ADB. 2020. *Public–Private Partnership Monitor, Indonesia. Manila.* https://www.adb.org/sites/default/files/publication/688886/public-private-partnership-monitor-indonesia.pdf.

89 OECD. 2012. *Indonesia - Public–Private Partnership Governance: Policy, Process and Structure. OECD Review of Regulatory Reform. Paris.* https://www.oecd.org/gov/regulatory-policy/Chap%206%20PPPs.pdf.

health security efforts and increasing health care system capacity throughout the pandemic.[90] Combined with external assistance and other contributions from civil society, it also resulted in relatively improved health security outcomes even during the worst parts of the pandemic in the country.

Lao People's Democratic Republic

Unique best practices in the Lao PDR remain limited, owing to its nascent PPP-enabling environment and the comparatively smaller impact of the pandemic in the country. However, the country's PPP Decree, enforced in January 2021, represents a step in the right direction as it systematically outlines the types of PPPs that can be pursued by the private sector and the procedures for doing so.

As in many countries, mobilizing the private sector boosted the public health care system capacity of the Lao PDR, given its existing resource constraints and infrastructure issues. On a donation basis, these PPPs provided crucial data management support, which was severely lacking, and helped boost both testing and vaccinations. Of the publicly available PPPs that materialized during the pandemic, two were related to the technological capacity of the private sector. One was the Lao Sou Sou app, a national effort to track COVID-19 infections and vaccinations. Collaborations between the public and private sectors allowed the country to leverage its capacity for innovation and roll out the app to monitor the national pandemic situation.

Overall, the experience of Lao PDR shows that an enabling piece of legislation can have a significant impact and that even donation-based PPPs can make a difference in upscaling capacity and stimulating innovation.

Philippines

The country has been emphasizing the role of PPPs in its national development strategy. The country's enabling environment is robust, with explicit, sector-specific laws and regulations related to national PPPs, public financial management, procurement, and social compliance in place.[91]

In response to the pandemic, the Government of the Philippines attempted to catalyze more PPPs in health care. One of the government's most prominent actions that serve as best practice in this regard was the Department of Health's establishment of a PPP for Health Program, a unit aimed at facilitating and optimizing PPPs in the health sector toward the development of health infrastructure and services.[92] Within this program, the Philippines has released a policy brief on "streamlining identification, development, and approval of PPP projects for the Department of Health," outlining a five-point intervention to guide the process of attaining PPPs in consultation with relevant health care stakeholders.[93]

---

[90] S. Preuss. 2020. Indonesia and COVID-19: What the World Is Missing. *The Diplomat*. 24 April. https://thediplomat.com/2020/04/indonesia-and-covid-19-what-the-world-is-missing/.

[91] ADB. 2018. *Public–Private Partnerships to Promote Transparency*. https://publications.iadb.org/publications/english/document/Public-private-Partnerships-to-Promote-Transparency.pdf.

[92] Government of the Philippines, Department of Health. 2021. Public–private Partnership for Health Program. https://doh.gov.ph/health-programs/Public-private-Partnerships-for-Health-Programs.

[93] H. Peña et al. 2021. *Streamlining Identification, Development, and Approval of PPP Projects for the Department of Health*. https://doh.gov.ph/sites/default/files/health_programs/Streamlining%20identification%2C%20Development%20and%20Approval%20of%20PPP%20projects%20for%20the%20DOH.pdf.

The Deputy Executive Director of the PPP Center also released a statement on investing in PPPs for health, outlining the types of PPP project structures in health care that the private sector could initiate, and the relevant agencies tasked with implementation.[94] This central focus on PPPs in health care, complemented by political will at the national level and with explicit guidance outlined, is arguably a vital best practice in ensuring more PPPs in health service delivery for the country in the near future.

The engagement model of the PPPs in the country during the pandemic has been unique. The government's call for private sector engagement to respond to the pandemic led to the creation of Task Force T3—a multisectoral public–private group of companies and organizations—that eased collaboration with the private sector in attaining HSI goals. Helmed initially by a handful of companies and public authorities to improve RT-PCR testing capacity, this partnership eventually expanded to include most of the country's business community. The efforts under Task Force T3 tackled all aspects of the pandemic response, including public vaccine education, vaccine incentivization, and personal protection equipment provision, among others.[95]

Moreover, PPPs during the pandemic were eased via coalitions such as the Philippines Disaster Resilience Foundation (PDRF), the country's primary private sector vehicle and coordinator for disaster risk reduction. This helped mobilize a network of private sector corporations, driving action in public education on vaccines in collaboration with other existing PPP campaigns such as the Ingat Angat Bakuna Lahat program.[96] In this light, Task Force T3 and the PDRF's Project K3 are examples of best practices in engaging the private sector on a broader scale during the pandemic while reducing the bureaucratic roadblocks of usual PPPs.

As also discussed in Chapter 2, the role of the private sector in communicating vaccines and countering hesitancy also deserves to be highlighted.[97] To dispel mistrust toward the government on issues related to vaccination, the private sector banded together to create vaccination campaigns, including incentivizing customers who got vaccinated. While not a sustainable long-term measure, this can also be considered a best practice in responding quickly to a public health crisis, with the private sector helping disseminate public health information on behalf of the state.

Thailand

The country stands out among the countries analyzed in this chapter. Despite being the first country outside the PRC to report a case of COVID-19, its adept management of the pandemic highlights the importance of a whole-of-society mobilization to meet shared objectives. While Thailand's success can be attributed to public sector initiatives such as its universal health care and the strength of its community volunteer programs, the private sector played a critical role during trying times.

---

94 PPP Centre. PPP Sectors. https://ppp.gov.ph/ppp-sectors-2/.

95 R. Bernardo. 2022. PPPs–Partnerships Towards a Progressive Philippines. *Business World.* 1 May. https://www.bworldonline.com/opinion/2022/05/01/445651/ppps-partnerships-towards-a-progressive-philippines/.

96 PDRF. 2021. PDRF Project K3 Recognized by COVID-19 Task Force; Continues Support to National Vaccination Program. News Release. 23 February.

97 A. Amit et al. 2022. COVID-19 Vaccine Brand Hesitancy and Other Challenges to Vaccination in the Philippines. 2 (1). pp. 1–23. https://journals.plos.org/globalpublichealth/article?id=10.1371/journal.pgph.0000165.

Thailand's foremost exemplary practice is having a clear and comprehensive PPP framework. As a result of iterative improvements over the decades, the country's PPP philosophy gradually developed from one broadly applicable and unclear to one focused on investment facilitation, with transparency and clear requirements, roles, and responsibilities integrated into it. When the pandemic hit, this framework allowed for faster response rates.

When the pandemic struck, existing PPPs were leveraged immediately, such as those between local governments, Ending Pandemics and OpenDream, and between Chulalongkorn University and Baiya Phytopharm, resulting in the creation of the PODD contact-tracing app and the Chula COVID-19 Test Strip Service. The construction of a new factory dedicated to manufacturing N95 face masks was funded by the private sector, ensuring a steady, free supply of masks for health care facilities and the general public during the early months of the pandemic. By the end of July 2020, 28 surgical mask factories were operating in the country, producing 4.2 million masks daily.[98]

Thailand's whole-of-society approach helped facilitate the logical solutions the pandemic required. During the worst COVID-19 surges, the country experienced bed shortages in quarantine centers, hospitals, and critical care units. However, through PPPs, hotels with minimal occupancy were repurposed for isolation and quarantine purposes, while private hospitals with critical care capacity (e.g., intensive care beds and airborne infection isolation rooms) stepped in to boost capacity. As the public health care system struggled to cope with the increasing case numbers, the government also collaborated with private health care providers in implementing the Universal Health Care Coverage Scheme while halving the claims submission period to every 15 days.

Finally, the involvement of public academic institutions in PPPs can be considered a third-best practice. It was one reason why Thailand managed to seize key economic opportunities during the pandemic, including involvement in vaccine research and development, trial, and manufacturing stages. The partnership between Chulalongkorn University and Baiya Phytopharm, a start-up company under Chulalongkorn University, encapsulated the potential of PPPs between public universities and pharmaceutical companies. Baiya Phytopharm has become the country's first pharmaceutical company capable of manufacturing medicines and vaccines from start to finish and was expected to be making its own COVID-19 vaccines publicly available by the middle of 2023.[99]

Timor-Leste

The country has a relatively small private health sector, in part because public health services are free at point-of-care and a comparatively small population that can afford to pay for private health care. In turn, public–private collaboration both before and during the pandemic has been limited, despite the country's numerous attempts to engage the private sector.

98 National News Bureau of Thailand. 2020. More Mask Factories Opened, Boosting Production Output to 4.2 Million Daily. 7 July. https://www.siamnews.net/business/25028-more-mask-factories-opened-boosting-production-output-to-4-2m/?amp.

99 *Bangkok Post*. 2022. Medicinal Marvel. 13 January. https://www.bangkokpost.com/business/2246803/medicinal-marvel.

Timor-Leste has worked with external knowledge partners and multinational development agencies to improve its PPP landscape. Before the pandemic, the country legislated a PPP law (Decree Law 42/2012) and established a dedicated PPP unit in the Ministry of Finance, overseen by the Council of Ministers. Through these efforts, as well as support from multinational agencies like the International Financial Corporation, the country managed to finalize its first PPP via a competitive tender in 2019, the Tibar Bay Port.[100]

Although Timor-Leste's enabling and regulatory environment for PPPs has a long way to go, the initial steps in establishing dedicated PPP governing institutions and legislation have constituted progress in driving greater public–private collaboration. In particular, the country's partnership with external knowledge partners has proven to be instrumental in improving the national PPP environment. These efforts to improve the PPP environment before the pandemic likely played a minor role in helping the government work with the private sector during the pandemic.

When COVID-19 hit, the government made efforts to tap the private sector to provide additional capacity and support public health efforts in testing, vaccine delivery, and quarantine measures—even as these public–private collaborations were small, informal, and sporadic, and despite the traditional lack of involvement of the private sector in health security. As COVID-19 cases rose and demand for vaccines, rapid testing, and quarantine facilities ballooned, the private sector continued to play a modest supporting role.

Stakeholder interviews for this chapter indicated that private hotels were converted into temporary quarantine facilities, private health clinics provided rapid testing for those who could afford it, and the very small private vaccination program helped deliver vaccines to about 1,000 people in the country. This, along with government efforts to leverage private sector networks for the delivery of essential social services during the emergency through a food basket program, demonstrated how the government's willingness to collaborate with the private sector, and vice versa, could still yield dividends for public health.

Recommendations

For Governments

Establish a Comprehensive Legal Regime for Public–Private Partnerships

PPPs offer tremendous benefits to both the public and private sectors. However, a comprehensive legal regime is crucial, especially because PPPs require long implementation periods and, at times, involve undertaking what is commonly seen as the state's responsibility by the private sector. A legal regime that outlines timelines and demarcates areas of authority, responsibility, and liability while ensuring

[100] I. Chatterton. 2019. *2018 IJGlobal Asia Pacific PPP Deal of the Year: Tibar Bay Port in Timor Leste.* https://www.unescap.org/resources/public-private-partnerships-infrastructure-development-primer.

transparency and information will enable PPP projects to be implemented smoothly. This legal regime should include a regulatory framework and strategy documents to attract more PPPs, as well as jurisdictional preference or alternative dispute settlement mechanisms to provide specific pathways for settling disagreements.

Furthermore, a comprehensive legal regime is also necessary because it removes the complexities associated with general investment or development laws that governments with nascent PPP frameworks usually apply to guide PPP projects. These are not considered good practices as laws are usually scattered across many legal instruments that risk increasing transaction costs. These general laws include, but are not limited to, those on private contracts, companies, taxation, labor, competition, consumer protection, insolvency, infrastructure, property, foreign investment, intellectual property, environmental, public procurement, and acquisitions and appropriations.[101] A strong legal regime and regulatory framework for PPPs simplifies procedures and facilitates more PPPs in the future. Overall, a comprehensive legal regime will ensure that the rights of both the public and private parties will be protected when entering into a PPP, helping bolster investor confidence.

Introduce Clear Public–Private Partnership Policy Frameworks

The length of PPP projects usually differs by type, with typical infrastructure projects spanning anywhere between 25 and 30 years.[102] This ensures that the investor can fully amortize the significant initial investment. This also places critical importance on prioritizing PPP projects to ensure that projected benefits are realized and projects are sustainable.

Long-term strategic plans outlining priority areas for PPPs can help achieve this end. For the private sector, these long-term plans can also serve as a means of promotion by highlighting various PPP opportunities, thus contributing to investment opportunities.

Clear policy frameworks can also outline requirements for the bidding phase, with bids subjected to a comprehensive analysis of socioeconomic viability and rigorous technical, financial, economic, and social feasibility. Wider national policy imperatives, such as those relating to environmental protection, can also be reflected in the bidding requirements. Taken together, these will ensure that despite the potentially differing interests and objectives of the parties, the PPP projects undertaken are sustainable from business, economic, social, and environmental perspectives.

Additionally, policy frameworks can integrate elements of good governance, such as transparency in the bidding, contract award, and implementation phases. This can help governments in their approach toward unsolicited PPP proposals that may be less competitive relative to a proper official selection procedure or, at worst, open up opportunities for corruption and abuse of power.[103] In many ways, such policy frameworks can keep both the public and private sector bodies involved accountable.

---

101 UNESCAP. A Primer to Public–Private Partnerships in Infrastructure Development. https://www.unescap.org/ttdw/ppp/ppp_primer/111_why_special_ppp_laws.html. Accessed 14 June 2022.

102 World Bank. Concessions Build-Operate-Transfer (BOT) and Design-Build-Operate (DBO) Projects. https://ppp.worldbank.org/public-private-partnership/agreements/concessions-bots-dbos.

103 World Bank. Unsolicited Proposals. https://ppp.worldbank.org/public-private-partnership/ppp-overview/ppp-procurement-bidding/unsolicited-proposals/unsolicited-proposals.

Through this balanced approach toward unsolicited PPP proposals, governments will be fully able to leverage private sector innovativeness toward problem-solving by widening the range of potential solutions while ensuring that public health goals remain paramount. While rigorous feasibility studies should be a prerequisite for any potential PPP project, this requirement is essential for unsolicited proposals where the private party might not be able to fully assess or appreciate the risks borne by the government. A well-designed policy framework governing unsolicited proposals should emphasize rigorous feasibility studies by a competent neutral party to ensure that the project is genuinely beneficial to the public interest.

Establish a Dedicated Agency Responsible for Public–Private Partnerships and Multi-Stakeholder Coordination

PPPs usually involve multiple stakeholders across all stages, from the needs identification stage to the project implementation stage. Coordination is critical in ensuring that interests and objectives are aligned, processes are streamlined, and overall coordination costs are minimized. This role is best performed by a dedicated government unit in the form of a permanent agency or ad hoc special-purpose vehicle that serves as a strategic platform for attracting and overseeing all PPPs. These agencies can also be tasked with drafting PPP policies, developing PPP expertise and knowledge, and advising government entities on adherence to PPP laws and best practices. Institutionalizing PPP expertise through these agencies can ensure the timely creation of constant improvements to the PPP legal regime and policy frameworks, with the country able to continuously improve its enabling environment.

These coordination bodies can contribute to the private sector in project implementation by facilitating the processes for applying for licenses and permits from various government agencies, as well as the issuance of the necessary approvals and authorizations. In doing so, these coordination bodies will be able to reduce the bureaucracy typically associated with PPP projects.

Create Multi-Stakeholder Consultative Processes

While PPPs can enable greater investment to meet urgent infrastructure needs, without a strong enabling environment, comprehensive legal regime, and clear policy frameworks, resource-poor countries will remain restricted in their ability to attract more PPPs. For developing countries, establishing multi-stakeholder consultative mechanisms can help support domestic efforts to gradually improve a country's PPP-enabling environment and institutional capacity.

These consultative mechanisms must include knowledge partners and multilateral development banks with deep expertise on PPPs, development partners, legal experts, relevant policymakers, business and investment councils, private sector stakeholders, and civil society. This will allow governments intent on introducing PPP laws and policies to fully appreciate the interests of the multiple stakeholders that may become eventual PPP partners, to learn from past and best practices of others, and to identify what potential partners may want to make PPPs viable and attractive to them.

Decentralize Public–Private Partnership Planning and Approval

Because PPP projects are typically large, they are usually planned, approved, and managed by central governments—sometimes at the cost of smaller, subnational PPPs. To this end, by decentralizing PPPs, subnational governments will be able to leverage the benefits of private sector participation in delivering public services.

With a coherent, overarching national development plan, the decentralization of PPPs can be made exclusive to specific sectors that could benefit the most from subnational planning. Administratively, PPP planning can be decentralized to state, provincial, and municipal governments. Meanwhile, the authority to approve PPP projects need not be decentralized to the smallest unit of subnational governance but rather can be vested in a competent authority at the highest subnational level. This will strike a balance between obtaining the benefits of PPP decentralization and maintaining oversight of potential decentralized PPP projects.

In conjunction, subnational governments can be allowed to determine PPP funding mechanisms—for example, through funding or credit guarantees from the federal or central government in combination with private sector funding. Politically, any effort toward decentralization of PPPs must be matched by high levels of transparency, good governance practices, and oversight mechanisms to mitigate risks of local-level corruption. Central or federal governments that are more experienced with PPPs must build capacity and share best practices with subnational governments. Efforts toward decentralization should also be done gradually rather than abruptly to ensure that subnational governments can cope with their increased responsibilities.

Align Domestic Public–Private Partnership Concepts with International Standards

By definition, PPPs involve multiple stakeholders, which means that each component may understand the objectives, roles, and responsibilities differently. This can pose barriers and challenges to understanding the needs of the procuring party and any subsequent bidding and negotiation, especially when it comes to foreign private companies. Aligning domestic PPP concepts and terminologies with those used internationally can help streamline processes, reduce time and effort, and boost the attractiveness of PPP opportunities. However, international standards should be adapted to local contexts.

Pursue Innovative Public–Private Partnership Projects to Further Unlock Value

Most PPPs have been in traditional infrastructure projects such as power and energy generation and critical transport links like roads and airports. Yet, the pandemic has highlighted the innovative potential of PPPs (e.g., in digital technology). Four of the six DMCs analyzed in this chapter created a mobile app that assisted with contact-tracing efforts during the pandemic. Building on the current momentum of PPPs in the health care sector, partnerships in telehealth and telemedicine, remote patient monitoring, digital therapeutics, and smart home technologies for caretaking must be given further weight and consideration.

PPPs in health care can also further utilize technologies such as big-data analytics for hospital staffing, electronic record keeping, real-time alerts, enhanced patient engagement, and strategic planning. Future PPPs should harness the innovative and dynamic capacity of the private sector and build more advanced systems and solutions. Legal and policy frameworks should be updated to ensure that the health care and other non-typical sectors ripe for PPPs can benefit from private sector participation.

Moreover, innovations must be considered to make companies planning to undertake or are undertaking PPP projects more attractive to investors. For example, private investment in public equity offerings where private investors are afforded an opportunity to purchase restricted stock at a more favorable price than is being offered to the public can make these companies more financially secure to undertake PPP projects.[104] This can be especially beneficial to PPP infrastructure projects undertaken through build–operate–transfer, where returns on investment are spread out over the long term. Private investment in public equity offerings can also benefit small- and medium-sized public companies that may have difficulty accessing more traditional forms of equity financing to bid on PPP projects.

Introduce Agility to Public–Private Partnerships During Times of Crisis

The novel and immense challenges of the pandemic highlighted the importance of introducing agility in mobilizing whole-of-society responses, particularly in public–private collaborations and PPPs. Examples include the Task Force T3 in the Philippines, the facilitation of private health care providers' claims for patient services in Thailand, and the private vaccination drives that contributed to the relative success of many countries' vaccination programs.

In terms of fully leveraging the contributions of PPPs in times of crisis, a balance must be struck between agile decision-making, reducing bureaucracy, and fast-tracking approvals while simultaneously ensuring the sustainability of PPP projects. One way to attain this is through special-purpose platforms that can coordinate PPPs during times of crisis. Incorporating open engagement models that allow public and private partners to communicate and collaborate freely can result in faster responses to urgent issues.

For the Private Sector

Augment Public Health Efforts—Not Just Health Care

As country experiences with the pandemic have shown, private sector health services work best when they complement and supplement existing government health security efforts. PPPs should increase capacity for responding to these urgent public needs. In the DMCs analyzed, the private sector actors involved tended to focus on specialized services that added to public health measures focused on primary preventative services. Similarly, private sector health care providers also augmented public health efforts by acting as spare surge capacity during sudden demand shocks, thereby playing a crucial role in the national pandemic response.

In this respect, there is a clear distinction between public health and health care. Public health activities address public health concerns like disease control, public education, and population nutrition. Health care activities involve health professionals like doctors and nurses delivering surgeries, medicines, and tests in clinics or hospitals. Traditionally, the private sector is involved in health care because of its size and potential profits; however, the private sector should consider public health efforts as a potential emerging market.

Help Increase Transparency and Accountability

In most countries analyzed, the lack of accountability and transparency concerning PPPs posed a significant barrier to more effective public–private collaboration. This barrier included a lack of clarity on how PPP projects were negotiated, finalized, and implemented. To hold public sector actors more accountable, the private sector can improve corporate governance,

---

104 T. Segal. 2022. What is Private Investment in Public Equity (PIPE)? Investopedia. https://www.investopedia.com/terms/p/pipe.asp#citation-2.

undertake periodic governance audits, and commit to transparency and integrity programs. This response will entail implementing robust compliance programs that conform to existing international standards, such as the G20/Organisation for Economic Co-operation and Development Principles of Corporate Governance (footnote 91). Likewise, mandating anti-bribery clauses in contracts related to public procurement projects and conforming to integrity pacts can create a more transparent business environment that benefits private businesses and governments.[105]

Drive Public–Private Dialogue Through Open Engagement Models

Beyond regular private engagement by governments, the private sector should also endeavor to improve public–private dialogue. Country experiences during the pandemic suggest that this form of engagement is most effective when done through open models where groups of companies and business leaders come together and leverage existing business networks like chambers of commerce to engage the government in areas of mutual interest. Through these institutions, the private sector can play a more direct role in communicating information and expertise and driving dialogue on potential avenues for public–private collaboration, ultimately reducing the transaction costs of bureaucratic and time efforts that traditionally impede the success and effectiveness of PPPs.

Move from One-Off Philanthropy Initiatives to Embracing Inclusive Development

The earlier analysis of the six countries revealed many instances of public–private collaboration taking the form of one-off donations or philanthropic contributions by private companies or individuals. While one-off donations doubtless helped improve health outcomes during the pandemic, there is certainly room for the private sector to go beyond such donations and impact their country's development more directly. This can mean integrating inclusive and sustainable development ideals into their core values and committing to contributions toward longer-term country development.[106] In integrating philanthropic and corporate social responsibility initiatives more closely with core business practices, private companies will be able to better align their goals with those of their national governments. Overall, this approach can enable more sustainable and longer-term public–private collaboration and dispel perceptions that private sector efforts to assist public service delivery are simply marketing strategies (footnote 106)."

For Multilateral Development Banks and Donors

Work with Developing Member Countries to Continuously Improve Public–Private Partnership Frameworks

For developing countries, the PPP regulatory and institutional environment will be a constant work in progress, incrementally improving as institutional capacity increases and economic development progresses. At the same time, DMCs in differing stages of development require different specific assistance in improving their PPP-enabling environment—with less-developed countries like Timor-Leste requiring closer end-to-end guidance from

---

[105] Transparency International. *Integrity Pacts—Civil Control Mechanism for Safeguarding EU Funds.* https://www.transparency.org/en/projects/integritypacts.

[106] OECD. 2011. *The Role of the Private Sector in the Context of Aid Effectiveness. Consultative Findings Document Final Report.* https://www.oecd.org/dac/effectiveness/47088121.pdf.

multinational development agencies in securing their first PPP agreement.[107] As such, DMCs will benefit from multilateral agencies taking an incremental and longer-term approach to capacity building in relation to PPPs.

Prioritize the Local Private Sector in Developing Member Countries when Delivering Assistance

Country experiences during the pandemic highlighted that assistance and aid from external donors and multilateral agencies worked best when their implementation involved local businesses and civil society organizations. For many less-developed DMCs, the lack of private sector dynamism was a major impediment to better public–private collaboration. When delivering assistance and aid, the donor community should involve and support domestic businesses and work with existing local networks like national and regional chambers of commerce. Additionally, external donors and development agencies could also highlight capacity building and knowledge transfer for involved local companies as key priorities in the delivery of aid and assistance. These efforts can lead to more sustainable and inclusive development in DMCs, besides improving the long-term capacity of the domestic private sector.

Contribute to Reducing Financing and Risk Gaps in Public–Private Partnerships

Multilateral development agencies and the donor community can help DMCs overcome two key barriers hampering greater public–private collaboration and PPPs: gaps in financing and the fact that PPPs in DMCs carry higher investment risk premiums for private partners and investors.

To that end, development agencies can not only directly contribute to financing PPPs; they can also play a role in reducing borrowing and transaction costs and investment risks for partner DMCs and private sector actors.[108] This can be through loan guarantees by multilateral development agencies, which can help gather private funds, reduce sovereign bond spreads, and increase bond tenures for high-risk developing countries. For instance, a 2007 World Bank loan guarantee for Bujagali Hydroelectric Plant in Uganda reduced the financing spread by about 5% and increased loan terms to 16 years.[109]

Multilateral agencies can also explore innovative financing mechanisms such as multidonor, co-funding lending, or guarantee arrangements. In 2015, ADB entered into a pilot co-financing agreement with the Swedish International Development Cooperation Agency to provide technical assistance, loans, and grants for numerous projects in Asia and the Pacific.[110]

---

[107] IFC. n. d. *Timor-Leste: Tibar Bay Port.* https://www.ifc.org/en/where-we-work/country/timor-leste (accessed 14 June 2022).

[108] M. Mohieldin et al. 2018. Multilateral Development Banks Must Mobilize Private Finance to Achieve the SDGs. *Brookings Institution.* 19 July. https://www.brookings.edu/blog/up-front/2018/07/19/multilateral-development-banks-must-mobilize-private-finance-to-achieve-the-sdgs/.

[109] P. Pereira dos Santos and M. Kearney. 2018. Multilateral Development Banks' Risk Mitigation Instruments for Infrastructure Investment. *Inter-American Development Bank. Office of Strategic Planning and Development Effectiveness Technical Note No. IDB-TN-1358.* https://publications.iadb.org/en/multilateral-development-banks-risk-mitigation-instruments-infrastructure-investment.

[110] ADB. 2015. *ADB Official Cofinancing with Sweden.* https://www.adb.org/sites/default/files/publication/159936/cofinancing-sweden.pdf.

Similar partnerships between multilateral development agencies and the wider donor community can mobilize more funding for projects and circumvent capital-treatment constraints faced by multilateral development banks (footnote 109).

Conclusion

This chapter offered an overview of health security intervention PPPs and public–private collaboration undertaken in six DMCs during the COVID-19 pandemic. The major finding is that DMCs with strong enabling environments in the form of comprehensive PPP legal regimes and policy frameworks, coupled with strategic PPP goals and political commitment at the national level, allowed for greater, faster, and higher quality PPPs to be created. These efforts helped turn some of the pandemic's challenges into economic opportunities. This is evidenced by the numerous PPPs on vaccine research and development, manufacturing, and distribution, which directly bolstered public health security efforts in the six countries.

Some countries used open engagement models to improve the agility of public–private engagement, moving away from typical PPPs (e.g., large-scale, long-term, heavily bureaucratic infrastructure projects). On the other hand, the countries with underdeveloped PPP legal and policy frameworks were still able to reap the benefits of PPPs, but the sustainability of their engagements remains questionable. As such, the key to attracting more PPPs lies in a solution long espoused by governments and multilateral development agencies: the improvement of PPP regulatory frameworks and enhancing the domestic regulatory environment. Such improvements are doubtless crucial to the swift delivery of effective responses in times of crisis.

Regardless of the differences in country experiences with private sector engagement during the pandemic, the six DMCs share one common need: greater investment in infrastructure, both within and beyond the health sector. The less-developed countries in the cohort are looking toward graduating from least-developed status in the coming years, likely leading to a corresponding decrease in external donor funding. By then, greater private sector collaboration and PPPs will become a key feature in recovering fully from the pandemic and accelerating economic development in the coming decade.

Overall, the pandemic has highlighted the fragility of existing systems, especially in public health. At the same time, it has emphasized the need for resilience and collaboration among all sectors of society. Responsibilities once intrinsically linked to the public health care system under the jurisdiction of the government (e.g., contact tracing, quarantines, vaccinations) have been complemented by the efforts of the local private sector, civil society, and the global donor community. Moving forward, it is necessary to create robust enabling environments where the interests of both public and private partners can be met. This means developing comprehensive legal systems that ensure the rights of all parties, as well as clear policy frameworks that highlight priority areas and opportunities for public–private partnerships. The opportunities to leverage the best attributes of the private sector in building more resilient and secure health systems run aplenty.

APPENDIX 1

Epidemics and Public Health Bureaucracy: A Conversation with Ly Sovann

Ly Sovann is the Director of the Communicable Disease Control Department of the Ministry of Health (MOH), Cambodia. The following is an edited transcript of an interview on 11 August 2023 via Zoom.

Cambodia does not have its own vaccine research center nor a self-sufficient vaccine manufacturing industry. Yet, the country was able to implement a relatively successful COVID-19 vaccination program. How were you able to do that?

Political commitment from the government is very important. Luckily for Cambodia, the government has always trusted us [its scientists and health experts] ever since the SARS outbreak of 2003, the avian influenza epidemic of 2009, and now COVID-19. We have always told the government that the quicker we respond to disease outbreaks, the earlier we can open up our country [after lockdowns]. Throughout COVID-19, whatever we recommended— "we" meaning not only my department, but also our partner organizations like WHO—the government followed. At first there was some confusion over what to do, of course, but eventually, all our government ministers learned to trust us.

When the government asked us [MOH] what the best bullet will be to control COVID, we said vaccines. That was how the government was able to prepare early in terms of importing vaccines from the PRC and the UNICEF's vaccine program. Hopefully, in future pandemics, vaccination will still be a priority for the government. It will be a new government by then, but most of its members would have worked closely with the MOH during COVID-19, so I do not think the policy will be changed.

We have spent more than $3 billion for our pandemic response. That includes major contributions, at least $100 million, from the private sector. We made the private sector understand that if we could not control the pandemic, businesses will surely collapse. It is very important to build trust between the government and the public. I can say that we have built this trust in Cambodia. Whatever we posted on our website and Facebook page, the people really trusted.

For rural areas, we had mobile teams that reached out to people who worked in remote agricultural industries and those who lived in the forests. Since we did not have enough vaccines at the time, we used the single-dose Johnson & Johnson [Janssen] vaccines for them, so we did not have to worry about their second doses.

Now for older people, we made a policy where we paid $250 to those older than 80 years old who would get vaccinated. That was how we were able to encourage our older populations to get vaccinated, which is why we have very high coverage among them.

Speaking of the SARS epidemic of 2003 and the avian influenza epidemic of 2009, how different was it back then compared to now with COVID-19?

During SARS, we did not have the response network that we have now. We started building this network only after SARS, in time for the avian flu of 2009. Back then, we were focused only on tackling priority diseases like tuberculosis, malaria, HIV, and dengue fever. We did not have early warning systems for emerging diseases. We also did not have the laboratory capacity or the logistical capacity for a vaccine cold chain.

Now, with the kind of network that we have and the kind of trust between the government and experts, we can initiate policy recommendations that would reach the prime minister in just 3 hours. At the start of COVID-19, it took us less than 24 hours to decide to lock down the country.

Moving forward, what do you think are the parts of the government response to COVID that need improvement?

One important thing is to allot funds for response teams to contain a disease outbreak at the site of the outbreak. This includes support to verify the possible outbreak. If you hear of a possible outbreak, you have to go to the community and verify it now, even if the information turns out to be false. Better to spend $50,000 on verifying outbreaks than millions of dollars on containing them at a much later time. I call this "emerging financial mechanism." For example, with dengue fever or measles, you do not wait for the outbreak to be big or visible enough to start responding. You have to actively look for people with a rash characteristic of dengue or measles in the community, or destroy breeding sites of larvae. You have to see all of it by yourself, with your own eyes, not just through someone's phone. When I was young, I would actually do this, go to the community to confirm the possible outbreak myself, but I was spending my own money. The funding then was only for containing outbreaks, not verifying them.

We also spend so much time and resources on bureaucracy—lots of money to follow bureaucratic guidelines on doing things, sitting down and talking, signing documents. Not just Cambodia, but the world. We are too busy with bureaucracy, which can be an obstacle to financial mechanisms meant for disease outbreaks. Now, I do it differently. If something is wrong, I tell my team to go immediately to the site of the possible outbreak to confirm it, no need to first have my signature on documents like mission orders. Just go. I call this "emerging administrative mechanism." You cannot contain an outbreak by prioritizing signatures, mission orders, or permissions. I tell my team, just text me what you need to do; there is no need to write a formal letter.

The intervals between pandemics are getting shorter. We know we will have one every 10 years. We had one in 2009, then 2019, so we can expect the next one 5 years from now. We have invested a lot of money in delaying pandemics, but not a lot on detecting and responding immediately to outbreaks. So, just to recap, first, we need to make sure that the public and politicians trust the experts. Next, we need to solve this culture of administrative and bureaucratic hierarchy. Finally, we need to have special financial mechanisms for emerging diseases to stop outbreaks at their very sources. For COVID-19, Cambodia has spent $3 billion, but we can actually spend just $100,000 investing in our responses to emerging diseases.

APPENDIX 2

Coronavirus and the Climate: A Conversation with Bounserth Keoprasith

Bounserth Keoprasith is the Director General, Department of Planning and Finance of the Ministry of Health (MOH), Lao PDR. The following is an edited transcript of an interview conducted on 14 August 2023 via Zoom.

What are your thoughts regarding the intersection between the climate crisis and the post-pandemic health situation? What are the urgent issues within this intersection?

The intersection between the climate crisis and post-pandemic health situation continues to be complex, especially for the least developed and poorest countries where health care systems are weak, people have unequal access to care, and climate change has not been put at the forefront of the national economic development and health agenda.

The Lao PDR is a witness to that. The country continues to face major health risks associated with climate change, including diarrheal and mosquito-borne diseases, malnutrition, and other related medical conditions and mental health challenges. Health facilities are vulnerable to extreme weather events associated with climate change, such as floods and storms. Smaller health centers in remote areas are especially vulnerable to structural and non-structural damage caused by extreme weather events; the health care system has limited capacity to maintain access to adequate power and safe water during hazardous events, during which times there is increased demand. The lack of access to adequate care affects the household economy through ongoing morbidity, loss of income and productivity, and medical expenses, contributing to reduced economic mobility and long-term intergenerational effects.

Besides the associated diseases, we also need to look at the intersection from a broader well-being perspective on climate change and health, including [through the dimensions of] governance, education, safety, and the economy. If we don't put climate change at the forefront of global and national economic development and health agenda, health inequalities will continue to widen. We are already witnessing the widening of existing gaps, especially among vulnerable populations of women, children, and adolescents among those living in low- and middle-income countries who are not prepared to face the upcoming challenges of the climate crisis. In most cases, these populations and countries have contributed minimally to greenhouse emissions, so it is simply unfair that they have been and will be disproportionately affected by the crisis.

The COVID-19 pandemic reinforced the connections between climate change and population health and overall societal resilience. It highlighted the centrality of effective public health systems to the reduction of poverty and other societal inequities. Without proactive action to prepare for and manage the climate crisis, the burdens of ill health will increase in the coming decades, with sustained detrimental impacts. It is, therefore, a very urgent need for developed and less-developed country leaders and governments to work together to close the gap of health inequality and include universal health coverage into climate change responses, making health services accessible to all people in the community.

How is the Lao PDR trying to climate-proof its health sector?

Climate change mitigation and adaptation are a priority of the government of the Lao PDR. The government is committed to the implementation of laws and policies related to climate change adaptation and mitigation, which will also contribute to achieving the SDGs and the Ninth National Social Economic Development Plan, as well as sectoral plans. Under SDG 13, initiatives undertaken to address climate change issues are (i) ongoing revision of the National Strategy on Climate Change and the completed revision of the Nationally Determined Contribution; (ii) completed climate vulnerability assessment and risk mapping in 18 provinces; (iii) initiation of the National Adaptation Planning process; (iv) initiation of and preparation for the work on building resilient urban populations with ecosystems-based solutions in six cities of six provinces; and (v) completed drafting of the Emergency Response Plan 2021 for the Natural Resources and Environmental sector.

The MOH, with technical and financial support from international organizations, conducted the Climate Change and Health Vulnerability and Adaptation Assessment 2019 with technical and financial support from ADB, the Strategy on Climate Change and Health Adaptation 2018–2025, and Action Plan 2018–2020. The government has been trying to improve health sector capabilities to respond to increasing climate change impacts. The MOH has been working collaboratively with the WHO country office to finalize the Health National Adaptation Plan (HNAP); the recently published Nationally Determined Contribution includes sections on human health.

However, there remains a need to strengthen the health system to safeguard and improve community health outcomes amid the volatile climate crisis. Strengthening overall health system capacity to become climate resilient is a target goal of the Strategy on Climate Change and Health Adaptation 2018–2025. In 2019, the Lao PDR joined the project, "Building Resilience of Health Systems in Asian Least Developed Countries to Climate Change," alongside five other Asian countries. This is a 4-year project (from 2019–2023) funded by the Global Environment Facility and implemented by UNDP and WHO in collaboration with the MOH. The project aims to help the MOH strengthen health system capacity to adapt to the impacts of climate change and to strengthen institutional capacity to improve health sector planning and effective decision-making for climate resilience. The following are the country's priorities under this project:

(i) **Developing and investing in safe–clean–green and climate-resilient health facilities and systems** by reducing emissions and strengthening management systems and institutional capacities to effectively integrate climate risks and adaptation options in health sector planning and implementation.
(ii) **Developing and building the capacity of the health workforce,** including administrative capacities, to effectively integrate climate change adaptation into health interventions and improve surveillance and early warning systems.
(iii) **Strengthening and improving climate-resilient health service delivery** by focusing on improving the capacity of the disaster management system and upgrading the national guidelines on emergency disasters and the medical emergency system. In collaboration with the WHO and World Bank, the MOH has piloted a number of activities to ensure that health facilities and their staff are resilient to climate change impacts and able to continue delivering services as the climate crisis worsens. In particular, (a) the country has developed and adopted the "Climate Resilient Water Safety Plan" training modules across five provincial- and seven district water suppliers; (b) the water and sanitation for health facility improvement (WASH FIT) tool (used for making safe, clean, and green health facilities) has been developed in the Lao language, with training for its use provided to central-level trainers and implementation in 14 district hospitals across two provinces; and (c) health care waste management training has been conducted in eight district hospitals in two provinces, including the development of improvement plans, with follow-up monitoring and technical assistance.
(iv) **Approving HNAP,** improving domestic and international cooperation and knowledge exchange, and integrating the HNAP into the national adaptation planning process led by WHO and UNDP.

What can the rest of Southeast Asia learn from the efforts of the Lao PDR's MOH to incorporate environmental concerns in health programs?

The Lao PDR continues to work on incorporating environmental concerns in health programs by working with different government ministries and developmental partners at different levels, from central to local communities, by involving local and international aid organizations and stakeholders across various ethnicities and genders in the communities. Much of the MOH's work has been with different government ministries and developmental partners and based on strong leadership, commitment, and coordination among health, environment, public works, and transport ministries, as well as other sectors critical to implementing climate-related activities. The MOH's working partnerships with different government ministries and developmental organizations, including ADB, WHO, World Bank, and UNICEF, have led to the continuous exchange of knowledge and experiences with the Lao PDR's Association of Southeast Asian Nations and non-association neighbors.

Our government is entering the "super year" of sustainability through accelerated implementation of the SDGs, along with other global frameworks such as the Paris Agreement on Climate Change, the Sendai Framework for Disaster Risk Reduction, and the New Urban Agenda. Health is the cross-cutting issue among these global frameworks. To meet these commitments, the Lao PDR will need to set clear policy goals for implementation supported by fiscal commitments and developmental aids to build a more resilient yet sustainable health system.

People are generally more concerned about health than the environment. How can we better communicate the urgency of environmental issues, as well as their intersections with human health?

Environmental and health issues are inherently intertwined. Much can be gained from addressing environmental health systemically. Behavioral health has much to offer in the understanding and promotion of environmental health, as human behavior is its central aspect. Environmental and behavioral health both offer behavior change theory as well as systematic approaches to enhance our understanding and promotion of mitigation and adaptation behaviors. It is, therefore, crucial to use scientific evidence to improve people's understanding and awareness of climate change—a critical issue that poses several direct and indirect health risks that will likely be amplified as the climate crisis accelerates.

People's behavior is central to promoting environmental health. On the one hand, people can mitigate their adverse impacts on the environment by changing their behaviors. Mitigation behaviors can thus alleviate the human impact on the environment. On the other hand, people can avoid or reduce adverse health effects brought about by their environments by adapting to environmental issues. Awareness is key: for example, by increasing public awareness through social media campaigns or by motivating people to walk instead of taking a car, which will not only reduce emissions but also promote active lifestyles.

However, all this can be done only with strong leadership and commitment from the government, as well as good public health policy. In addition, investment in climate change and health adaptation, as well as stricter laws and policies regarding environmental health, will contribute to people's long-term behavioral changes and adaptation to the climate crisis.

APPENDIX 3

Legislation, Cooperation, Public Investment: A Conversation with Rattanaxay Phetsouvanh

Rattanaxay Phetsouvanh is the Director General, Communicable Disease Control Department of the Ministry of Health (MOH), Lao PDR. The following is an edited transcript of an interview conducted on 16 August 2023 via Zoom.

How is the health situation right now in the Lao PDR post-pandemic? What's on your mind right now in terms of the health care system?

We are facing the usual seasonal diseases. In fact, we are now facing a big dengue outbreak. Unlike COVID, where you have tests and vaccines, dengue remains challenging to manage, and because it's been around for so long, people are not as invested in following our recommendations. So, this is the dilemma if you compare to COVID-19. Of course, there are orders on diseases like seasonal flu. There are a lot of flu-like illnesses in the Lao PDR because of the typhoons that have come up post-pandemic.

What are the lasting benefits of the systems you put into place during COVID-19 for the public health system in the Lao PDR as we move beyond the pandemic?

One thing we learned from the pandemic was that our public health services were not ready. Even if we were prepared, the services were not well equipped. Buying time was what we ended up pursuing at the beginning. Unlike some of our neighbors, like Thailand or Viet Nam, our hospitals were not well-equipped, so we had to keep the country free from COVID until we had the tests, the drugs, and the vaccines.

To some extent, our interventions were successful, even though we had to face the challenge of accommodating Laotian migrant workers from different countries around the world. Most of these workers became jobless because the businesses they worked for collapsed. And in the countries they worked in, they were not treated as citizens. They didn't have enough support, like places to stay, food, or access to tests. Had we kept our borders closed from these migrant workers, it would have been controversial and damaging to the reputation of our public interventions. So, we allowed all these workers back into the country.

Legislation was crucial to our COVID-19 response, and it is critical to moving beyond the pandemic. When COVID struck, we had our communicable disease law, which was very good because if we didn't have this law, we would probably have faced difficulties. Under this law, there's a provision for a National Committee for Communicable Disease which allowed us to move forward efficiently as an organization.

We also learned the importance of social media, of receiving (and giving) feedback to people. Thankfully, we've had the time to review all of these now, I think, and we have already updated versions of our communicable disease law. It's very good, though there are a lot of things to improve, of course. I think there's no perfect legislation, but our new law anticipates challenges like funding sources and the role of the private sector, among others. We have also laid out the roles of different facilities: between private and public, at the individual, family, and community levels. So, the law is more comprehensive than before.

How can Southeast Asia prepare for the next pandemic?

A lot of countries were surprised to see the Lao PDR contain COVID-19 faster than them. But actually, it was not our strength alone; we worked with various partners. For example, we communicated with our Thai colleagues, "Could we get some tests ?" And they granted our request. We set up our surveillance system with PRC since we shared land borders. The public was also very supportive and understanding of our limited capacity, especially at the beginning of the pandemic. Of course, we also saw the increased role of health professionals, as well as those who had to work in the frontlines, including police officers. They are the ones who deserve the credit.

The health sector alone could not have solved the problem. This does not mean that other sectors could have done it by themselves; it's cooperation among all sectors that's key.
At the start, the private sector didn't want to contribute more than they should to the COVID response. So, a lot of people didn't go to the private hospitals. Not a lot of cases landed in private hospitals, which didn't want to help the public hospitals either. We had to improve this system through a free COVID-19 hotline in such a way that we could distribute the patient load more equitably among hospitals.

We also needed to have the trust of the public. If the public were with us, they would do what we recommended. So, cooperation is really key, both within our countries and across the region. Investing in the public sector should really be high on our list of priorities. Compared to before, we never thought that we could expand and improve our facilities, but it mattered a lot that we did. I believe continuing such investments will allow us to be better prepared for the next health crisis.

APPENDIX 4

Challenges and Lessons from Thailand: An Interview with Vichan Pawun and Chaninan Sonthichai

Vichan Pawun (VP) is the head of Thailand's Bureau of General Communicable Diseases. Chaninan Sonthichai (CS) is a Medical Officer, Department of Disease Control of the Ministry of Public Health, Thailand. The following is the edited transcript of an interview conducted on 27 September 2023 via Zoom.

Thailand was a big inspiration for many countries in terms of the overall success of your vaccination program. Looking back at what happened, especially at the beginning of the vaccine rollout, what do you think were the major reasons why Thailand had such a good program for vaccination?

VP: Vaccination might be the biggest task during a pandemic situation. In my opinion, the first challenge was the introduction of the vaccine during the pandemic. The vaccine that we used was under emergency use authorization. So, we had to balance between scientific information about the safety and the effectiveness of the vaccine. We had to communicate with the group of experts, but we also had to communicate with the people. So, we had to balance the safety data.

The second challenge was allowing the mechanism to get the vaccine during the pandemic. Because we didn't have a vaccine factory, we couldn't produce vaccines in Thailand, so we had to import from other countries. During the crisis, it was quite a challenge because we had to work closely with the government [and] the politicians because it's about vaccine negotiation between countries. So, we had to work with the higher levels of government to negotiate to get vaccines to Thailand.

The third challenge was the implementation. During the pandemic, we wished to keep vaccinations as much as possible to increase the covalence of the vaccine as much as possible. So, we had to activate all vaccination units. That included the public, private, and many units. During COVID, we convinced a big superstore to be part of our vaccination unit. For example, we had a mobile vaccination unit to go to the fresh market, to go to the temple, and to many places in the community to provide vaccinations.

The fourth challenge was the information system. We don't have strong infrastructure for IT or technology. [As] the public sector, we had to educate the private sector to build what we call a cloud system to develop the information system to get the data out on immunization. It was quite challenging, but we got good responses from the private sector to develop our system. Right now, we call it the OPS IC cloud system or MOC IC cloud system. And this system right now we are planning to develop to be part of our immunization program with the EPI vaccine or other vaccine. We can use this system.

CS: Because COVID vaccines were very new vaccines, we had to deal with both sides of the population. On one hand, those who preferred getting COVID vaccines, getting every shot, and on the other hand, some people were still concerned about the safety and efficacy of the vaccine. Again, this was partly because it was a new vaccine and different from the routine immunizations that we have implemented for a long time. So, for COVID vaccines, we had fake news, misinformation through social media, and we have had to work with our partners to respond to this misinformation to get the public to understand COVID vaccines.

Another challenge about COVID vaccines was that the scientific data were not enough in the early phase. So, we had to adapt our strategy to fit with the new data or the new findings from the research. And we had to communicate this evolving nature of scientific knowledge to the public.

In terms of communication—of communicating vaccine safety and convincing the public to get vaccinated—who were the other key actors you worked with?

VP: I think we have many layers to public communication. At the top level, at the government level, we have a specific committee. At the government level, they educate the ministry. And they have a spokesperson, and the spokesperson at that level is also a doctor. He is the secretary, so he can communicate with the general public. He is very, very good in teaching the message that we need to communicate through the program. So, the spokesperson at the government level, he was also a medical doctor. And at the implementation level, as Chaninan mentioned, we have this unit to monitor fake news. Once we detect something that we need to clarify, we have a group of experts with specialties, many experts on vaccines.

After discussing the issue in detail at the ministry level and the department, we would assign a spokesperson and also the doctor, who is very well known in the department, to communicate to the public. So, my point is that we don't do things alone; we have a group of experts that includes the experts in the academy, in the dual-state hospital, and people that we have to educate on clarifying the message before sending them out to the public. For the media side, I think the media in Thailand work fairly with the public health ministry. They have worked with us for a long time. So, when we have something that we have to clarify with the media, we would invite the media.

Were there particular groups that were challenging to communicate with? For example, in the United States, vaccines became a politicized issue. Was there any particular challenge that you faced in terms of a particular group in Thailand?

CS: The challenge is also the anti-vax group. We also have the anti-vax group. And, I don't know, they have data and share them with the public. And we have to change that. Not only the anti-vax group, but, in my opinion, there is also an anti-government group because the vaccines were issued by the government. So, this kind of discredit of the government is one of the many things that has happened to the vaccine campaign.

What is the possible role of regional cooperation for pandemic preparedness in the future?

VP: There are efforts within ASEAN to have a mandate for coordinating vaccine efforts, such as importation and acquisition; we also saw this happen during the Mpox [monkeypox outbreaks], in which Indonesia helped other member countries. So perhaps we are seeing the development of a regional mechanism; it is not a strong system yet, but it is a good starting point.

CS: Collaboration between countries is really a crucial mechanism to facilitate pandemic preparedness. I must add that, beyond the region, we need to work with various international organizations. If there's anything that the pandemic taught us, it is that one country cannot respond to the pandemic alone.

APPENDIX 5

Strengthening Local Institutions: A Conversation with Beverly Ho

Beverly Ho is Assistant Secretary of Health-Public Health Services of the Department of Health (DOH) of the Philippines. The following is the edited transcript of an interview conducted on 6 October 2023 via Zoom.

Much has been said about equity, the need to build trust, and the need to communicate to the public as far as COVID-19 vaccinations are concerned. As someone who's been in the midst of policymaking and implementation, what are the discourses surrounding vaccinations and the lessons we can learn from them that around lessons learned in vaccination, COVID vaccination?

What we've learned from the Philippine experience is that vaccination success is really related to access to services and the ease of accessing them. What we're seeing is that it's not just vaccine hesitancy. At the national level, you can tell people to get vaccines or to get vaccinated, but it seems like the issue at the local level is people not really knowing where to get the vaccine. In the United States, you can just walk into a CVS [pharmacy chain]; in other countries, you can go anywhere. I think the fragmentation of our local health system is a critical factor to this. At the national level, we can always announce a vaccine, but we never really achieved being able to tell the public where the actual sites were and what time they're open or closed.

I myself don't actually know where to point people since the national government just gives the vaccines to the LGU, and the national role ends there. In the end, it's still up to the LGU to decide how to make vaccines available, if there's only one health center where it will be available, or if they will set up dedicated vaccine clinics. It takes a lot of back and forth to get that information. Of course, you'd expect them to announce that information themselves, but again, it's up to each and every LGU and we don't have any control. So, overall, the fragmentation has been really a major barrier.

Within this variability, given the unevenness of this implementation at the LGU level, was there a pattern among LGUs that tended to perform better in terms of delivering vaccinations?

If you're a better-resourced LGU, it was really easy because you were also engaged in healthy competition. But even then, especially when we were scaling down the programs, it was still up to LGUs to decide what to do. If the goal now is to embed COVID-19 vaccination within existing immunization programs, then it becomes dependent on regular working hours, which in turn depends on each LGU's policies.

So, in a way, it's an equity issue on another level, not just at the level of individuals, but at the level of where people live. But do you think the pandemic brought a fresh realization that this is happening? And have there been steps to resolve this now that it's been laid bare for people to see that this is problematic?

But who will do this micro-planning? Isn't this solution also contingent on the unevenness of the system and the lack of LGU capacity?

I think one of the biggest takeaways after the pandemic is to revisit LGU performance and emphasize the importance of applying the concept of micro-planning to immunization programs. This entails attending not just to major things like procurement, but also minor yet crucial aspects like resources, supplies, forms, personnel, and, of course, data. At the end of the day, a rural health unit or a health center still needs to plan. For every 100,000 people you have, you need to know how many more are likely to come on a daily basis. It's really all about understanding and managing service delivery at the micro level.

In terms of communications, is there also any added value to these province-level health systems that can facilitate health communications, either specifically for vaccines or for health promotions in general?

True, but we can consolidate at the provincial level. So, you just need 80 big units to plan on behalf of the over 1,500 LGUs. At the provincial level, resources can be moved and reallocated around depending on the needs of specific municipalities instead of leaving them on their own. The Universal Health Care Law calls for developing province-wide health systems is an enabling mechanism for this direction, but it's a question of whether and how we will take this seriously.

In that sense, because of all the challenges we faced with COVID, we also saw the pathologies of the health system. Do you think there's a level of reflexivity on the part of the government to learn from these lessons?

Surely, and that's what we're hoping for: that there will be spillover effects. After all, vaccination is a tracer of all the basic services of the health system.

Yes, of course. We're modifying the LGU planning tools now because they're really not responsive. They don't have the granularity that's required for operational work. Part of it is really not just counting what frontline service inputs you need but institutional strengthening in terms of planning the delivery. What we've been reminded of is that there are many moving parts within the entire service delivery, and we need to plan accordingly.

This will require political will. During the COVID-19 public health emergency, we had unprecedented support from all sectors: private sector, government, and politicians. But now that the emergency is over, do you think there's still space to generate enough attention or action toward this kind of health systems strengthening? What are the challenges moving forward?

We just have to keep doing what we're doing. We may have faced challenges, but we've also had some gains; I think we're definitely much improved in terms of vaccine confidence. But we can't let our guard down. When it comes to public attitudes on vaccination, it's like walking on eggshells, especially when some medical practitioners themselves are against vaccination. And, of course, adverse effects are real. But when these stories of adverse effects are being used by anti-vaxxers, it becomes highly problematic. Still, we're in a better place than we were after the Dengvaxia [dengue vaccine] scandal.

We also saw the unprecedented contributions from the typically for-profit private sector, many of whom pitched in for different aspects of the vaccination effort, from procurement to communication. The challenge is to get them to continue their support, but these doors for collaboration have been opened.

All the things that others have emphasized are critical, but there has to be an infrastructure to make plans happen. At the end of it all, we have to acknowledge that we have a country that is so big and diverse, and it's just difficult to orchestrate 1,500 municipalities without capacitated, functioning local health systems. We really have to work toward institutional strengthening at the level of local government.

www.ingramcontent.com/pod-product-compliance
Lightning Source LLC
Chambersburg PA
CBHW041757220926
51847CB00014B/231
* 9 7 8 9 2 9 2 7 7 2 0 8 6 *